PARTY GOWN

a DOCTOR's LaUGHaBLe aDVICe

CATHERINE WOODHOUSE, MD

Party Gown: A Doctor's Laughable Advice

For information about this title or to order other books and/or electronic media, contact the publisher:
Poema Enterprises
PO Box 669482
Marietta, GA 30066
www.laughableadvice.com

Library of Congress Control Number: 2016947810

ISBN: 978-0-9967399-0-0 (Paperback)
978-0-9967399-1-7 (eBook)

Printed in the United States of America

Cover and Interior design: 1106 Design

Publisher's Cataloging-in-Publication
(Provided by Quality Books, Inc.)

Woodhouse, Catherine, author.
Party gown : a doctor's laughable advice / Catherine Woodhouse.
pages cm
LCCN 2016947810
ISBN 978-0-9967399-0-0 (pbk.)
ISBN 978-0-9967399-1-7 (e-book)

1. Patient education--Humor. 2. Physician and patient--Humor. 3. Medical care--Humor. 4. Humor. I. Title.

R727.4.W66 2016 613
QBI16-900021

TABLE OF CONTENTS

Disclaimer

This book is a work of humor. It presents general health information in an entertaining way.

This book is not meant to be used or relied on for any official diagnostic or treatment purposes, does not create any patient-physician relationship, and should not be used as a substitute for individualized professional diagnosis and treatment.

Please consult your physician or other qualified health care provider for any and all specific decisions or guidance regarding your own particular situation and concerns.

The Author, Poema Enterprises, and any other affiliates expressly disclaim responsibility, and shall have no liability, for any damages, loss, injury, or liability whatsoever suffered as a result of reading or following the information contained in this book. Reliance on any information in the book occurs solely at your own risk.

And please never disregard formal professional medical advice or delay seeking care because of something you read in this book.

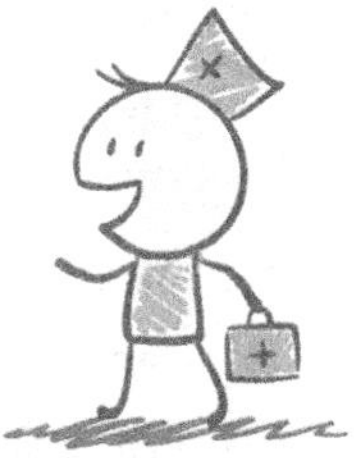

INTRODUCTION

SNAG RIPPLING ABS BY READING THIS BOOK

YES, YOU! HERE'S THE SECRET. Just balance this special book squarely on your belly. Then, while you're reading, do about five hundred sit-ups, and voilà! You will *definitely* feel your abs rippling.

Or, you can simply accept the substandard abs you already have and settle in for an interesting read. Yummy snacks are optional.

In these pages, I'm inviting you on an unusual excursion—a silly little jaunt through the medical universe. If you've ever been a patient or taken care of one, you already know the situations you can find yourself in are just plain weird, and the doctors are even weirder. Even in the midst of needing care, there are still lots of opportunities for laughter.

If you're a healthcare professional, you get to laugh at yourself too. A merry heart is good for the soul!

Together we'll chuckle our way through the doctor's office, the ER, and the hospital; explore common health concerns; shop for health insurance; and even get a peek at the future of medicine. I'll show you what your doctor is thinking so you can better understand any odd behavior you encounter. Lastly, you can discover how to have the best possible life *ever,* hands down.

I choose to use *physician, doctor,* or *doc* instead of the more recent term *provider,* which is meant to be inclusive of nurse practitioners and physician assistants. These advanced practitioners are productive, vital members of many medical staffs and hospitals and can provide excellent care. But *provider* is a stale, barren label for anyone, reducing medical care to an indifferent marketplace transaction. To all of my fellow colleagues, feel free to make any substitutions you see fit.

To all of you wonderful newbie and veteran patients: Please remember you're not alone, and try to laugh whenever you're able. To everyone: Enjoy!

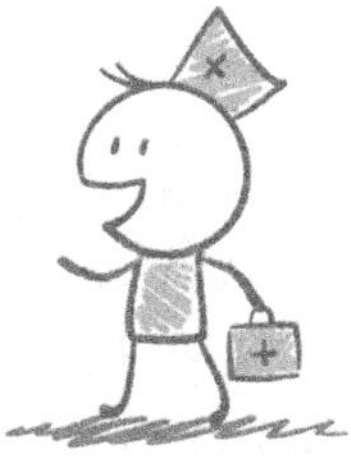

CHAPTER 1
STEERING CLEAR

Does an apple a day keep the doctor away?
If you aim it well enough.
—Anonymous

LET ME GUESS. You *hate* going to the doctor, right?

Imagine for a moment that you're being seen at the best medical practice ever created: Patient Paradise. Patient Paradise is wonderfully well run and renders superb care. There are no long waits, no embarrassing personal questions, and no drafty gowns. Your office visit, including blood work and all the very best tests, is totally free. Free. No bill. Patient Paradise also has a café with coffee, pastries, and sandwiches, full-body massage, auto detailing, and a stand-up comedian, all of which, again, are completely free.

Incredibly, you would still hate going. Most folks do.

What is it that makes most people want to chomp down as many apples as possible to try to keep the doctor away? When they do finally see a physician, they scramble frantically to flee with their dignity and wallets intact. That's why patients can't remember half of what doctors tell them—they're too busy plotting their escape while keeping half an ear open for a vague "you'll probably be okay" statement of some sort.

Whose fault is this? Mature and introspective professionals that we doctors are, we typically begin by shifting blame. But not in this book! Here, we doctors will take the first hit. How have we contributed to the general public's massive medical aversion?

Quite frankly, some of us are jerks.

Even going to nice doctors is usually painful, notoriously expensive, and incredibly inconvenient, and it may involve potentially lethal prescription drugs. These pesky annoyances aside, there are other important reasons why doctors are kept at arm's length.

The most prevalent is embarrassment. People don't make appointments because they worry their doctors will think badly of them. They worry, for instance, that we'll laugh when they tell us their entire weight-loss plan hinges on using a ThighMaster. (Yes, we will, but only for a brief second.)

Another common reason is: "I'm too sick to come in!" Doctors quite naturally have a very difficult time comprehending this one. Then there's the "My breath/feet/etc. stink," conditions which we wholeheartedly agree should be handled well before the appointment as much as humanly possible. Lastly, there are the people who view it as a huge personal failure to have to come in. When they are no longer able to beat back their illness solo, they drag in, apologizing for "wasting the doctor's time"—yet another odd reason to not go to the doctor.

But here's the catch: Seeing the doctor prior to something going terribly wrong might just help you avoid it. At least, we docs believe so. And it's not because we have a vested (read: financial) interest in seeing our patients' lovely faces; it's because we've seen the face of disease, and it's not pretty.

Prevention is key. Doing nothing to prevent disease is like trying to drive your car for a hundred thousand miles without ever changing your oil or inflating your tires. And unlike a car, you can't just go out and buy a new body. (At least, you can't yet.) You've got to make yours last as long as possible. Even if it's got three hundred thousand miles on it and it's making funny noises, it's not too late!

Let's find a doctor, shall we?

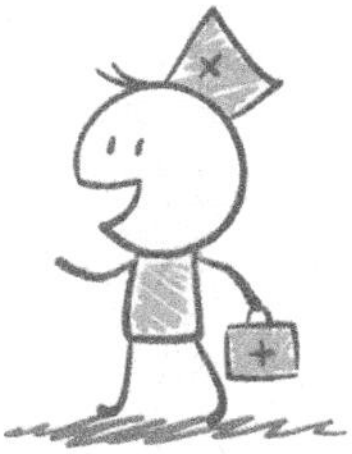

CHAPTER 2
FINDING A DOCTOR WHO ISN'T A FIEND

I become faint and nauseated during even very minor procedures, such as making an appointment by phone.

—Dave Barry

HOW DO YOU FIND a great doctor, especially if you're new to an area? Word of mouth works well. But if you need a proctologist, that might get tricky. What then?

Before the Internet, you would open the Yellow Pages and blindly select a physician whose last name sounded halfway competent, like "Dr. William Abramson III." These days, you visit your insurance company's website and blindly select a physician whose last name sounds halfway competent. Then you visit the state medical board's website to make sure that person is indeed a real doctor and that he hasn't killed anybody.

Are doctor-rating websites reliable? Well, it depends on how many computer-savvy patients take the time to post their opinion. Let's say Dr. White is an excellent family practice physician who has been in practice for ten years, enjoys great relationships with his patients and staff, and has never been sued. If only two of Dr. White's patients log in and post favorable comments, Dr. White gets a perfect score and looks like a rock star. However, if a single unhappy patient subsequently chimes in, Dr. White's once-golden rating nosedives like a shoddy paper airplane. Does that mean he's one step away from having his license revoked? Not at all. However, these websites can be useful to help you avoid truly malignant providers. One bad review is not the end of the world. Many bad reviews are worth paying attention to.

For me personally, the search for a physician is even harder. "But Dr. Woodhouse," you might say, "isn't it nice to be a doctor? When you get sick, you already know someone good to go to." Sure, but the problem is that I know the doctors professionally. I don't want them knowing my personal business too! And because their staff would be involved in my care too, there is ample potential for awkwardness:

Dr. Woodhouse (calling my personal doctor's office on behalf of a mutual patient): "Hello, this is Dr. Woodhouse. I need to speak to someone about working a patient onto Dr. Higgenbottom's schedule urgently, if you'd be so kind."

Receptionist (excitedly): "Oh, hi, Dr. Woodhouse! How *is* that hemorrhoid of yours?"

Dr. Woodhouse: "Uh . . ."

Receptionist (hollering loudly, alerting all the patients in the waiting area): Glenda, it's Dr. Woodhouse! Come talk to her about her hemorrhoid!"

Nurse Glenda (slyly): "Well, hello, Dr. Woodhouse—are you finally able to sit down these days?"

You get the picture. Knowledge of who the "really good" doctors are may be a pointless piece of information when it comes to my own care, unless I'm willing to abandon every ounce of pride. Or don an extremely good disguise.

Proper Office Recon

Once you've completed your doctor research, consider a bit of office reconnaissance before you finally commit to making an appointment. Avoid looking too conspicuous, or the staff will forever remember you as "that weird person" when you finally do come in.

The first thing you should assess is what's adjacent to the office. A medical office that backs up to a graveyard or funeral home is less desirable. Also, check out the signage. In an ideal world, the office would have a sign clearly stating its intentions. Even before you set foot inside, you would know that you needed to turn around and go back home. Some examples of bad signage:

Abandon All Hope Ye Who Enter Here

Your Money Or Your Life

Don't Call Us; We *Might* Call You

Park at Your Own Risk (Not Responsible for Theft-Robbery-Assault)

What about the building itself? Is it better to see a doctor who works in a posh, ultramodern office rather than one who works in a more modest one? Remember that office space equals overhead. The more classy the office, the more classy the overhead.

That overhead has got to be paid somehow, and most likely that would be by you.

Look for accommodations for the mobility challenged—ramps, automatic sliding doors, and railings. If they're sparse, it might mean that:

1. The doctor doesn't plan on seeing those patients (and you'd better watch how he treats you if you should sprain your ankle and end up on crutches);
2. Those patients, having suffered multiple nasty falls trying to get up the steps, will greatly assist the doctor in meeting his monthly overhead; or
3. The doctor is so fantastic that by the time those patients leave, they don't need any assistive devices.

The Waiting (and Waiting) Room

Let's assume that you find a decent doctor's office and that you've taken the leap of faith and scheduled your appointment. You take a deep breath and stride expectantly through the office door. What's your first impression? Is the office a pleasant haven of tranquility, or a scene from Armageddon? Is it a relaxing enclave, or a dingy debacle that looks remarkably like your own unkempt house on a really bad day? Are the chairs comfortable and clean, or are they sticky with crusted food? Are there just a few people quietly waiting to be seen, or does the waiting room look like an awkward sleepover, with sick people crowded together and strewn across the floor?

Next, visit the bathroom. Scented potpourri in handsomely decorated baskets is good. Unidentifiable material smeared on the walls is bad. Extra toilet paper, attractively displayed, is good. No toilet paper is bad. Trust me: If an office truly cares about the cleanliness of its bathroom, more than likely it will care about you. Pay attention to details. Are all the houseplants in the office dead? Little things do matter.

Assess the mood of the staff. This will tell you a lot about the office leadership. It is a red flag if the staff members visibly hate their jobs, hate their doctors, and hate each other. Your care will inevitably get caught up in the middle of all that negativity. Are the receptionists attentive and content? Or are they distracted and stressed out? Do they speak politely to patients on the phone? Or are they palpably annoyed?

How are the nurses? Their attitude can also give you important clues about how healthy an office is. Happy nurses tend to be well-cared-for nurses. Typically, really good nurses don't stay hooked up with really bad doctors—they just don't stand for it. And if the nurses have those little pointy hats on, run!

YOUR PAPERWORK

Paperwork is a necessary evil. Basically, the office wants to know who you are, and more importantly, who will pay the bill if you kick the bucket unexpectedly or become too incapacitated to write a legible check or whip out your credit card. It would be rather awkward if the staff had to reach into your wallet for you. (And you thought the "emergency contact" section was so the office could notify a loved one in case you had a medical problem!)

The office will want you to manually write out your insurance information, even though they've already made multiple copies of your insurance card and driver's license. This is so you can certify that you're not making anything up. Then you're given a medical history form so that you can share all your deeply personal health secrets. This provides the various staff members handling your paperwork with interesting reading material during their breaks.

Lastly, enter the HIPAA form. HIPAA stands for the Health Insurance Portability and Accountability Act. This government-mandated sheet of paper explains that your health information is supposed to be private. By signing this form, you acknowledge that unauthorized access to your personal information is illegal. Great! Since HIPAA was passed, I have been informed that my medical file has been compromised on three separate occasions. But thanks to my HIPAA form, I'm confident that each of the criminals will notify me before they engage in any illegal activity using my information.

The Exam Room

So far you've assessed the physical building, the waiting room, and the staff. You've been a good citizen and tried hard not to omit embarrassing information on your medical history form. Now you're waiting in the exam room, and more data about the suitability of your choice is available to you. How clean is the room? Has the exam-table paper been freshly changed, or is someone else's rear-end print still on it? Do you see the doctor's credentials framed prominently and elegantly, or is her diploma a grease-spotted, off-kilter, bad copy attached to the wall by a tack? Please don't worry if you see that your doctor was educated someplace you aren't familiar with. If I were you, I'd be more concerned about the copy/tack situation.

If You See a Bug

Several years ago, I was working down South, and in the midst of a lovely visit with an unbelievably sweet newlywed couple, the wife suddenly emitted a bloodcurdling shriek. I was sitting on my examination stool facing them with my back toward the exam-room sink. A gigantic, prehistoric bug had emerged from the overflow drain and was lunging in our direction. I jumped back to defend myself. This beast was *huge*. I had to run and get the nurse, because that's what we doctors do whenever we're in trouble: Get the nurse. It's in the doctor handbook.

After the nurse had called the local HAZMAT team to dispatch the creature, the idyllic office visit was decidedly over, and I never saw that unbelievably sweet couple again. Perhaps they thought I didn't have their best interests at heart because I abandoned them in the room and didn't ensure they were evacuated first. Perhaps they assumed that the office was less than hygienic. Perhaps they were scarred for life. But the office was not unhygienic, and we never saw a similar bug again. Barring a mutant insect threatening to gnaw on you and then take over the planet, you can probably rest easy if you see a bug in the doctor's office.

If You See Something Worse Than a Bug

I once served in a very old, tiny clinic near a downtown waterfront. My staff and I began to find small clumps of brown debris on our desks each morning. In my infinite doctorly wisdom, I assumed my desk was dusty. I would wipe off the "dust" with my hand every day before I started seeing patients (yet another reason to make absolutely sure that your doctor washes her hands before she touches you). My nurse at the time, who possessed way more common sense than I did, immediately knew there was something afoot (literally). But we were told repeatedly by higher-ups that there was no way rodents could possibly be in the building.

One day, I was smack-dab in the middle of doing a Pap smear when I heard the pitter-patter of little feet. Then I saw a rat scamper across the room and under the door. The patient, glancing distractedly around the room, said, "What was that noise?"

In the brightest singsong voice I could muster, I replied, "Oh, nothing," and finished up her exam as quickly as I could. I had another unfortunate rat encounter just a short while later when I was alone in the ladies' room. Needless to say, the vermin situation was rapidly handled after that point. As a general rule, if you're in the exam room and you see a living, breathing, flea-infested animal running amok, singing "Born Free," pass on that office.

Other Concerning Things in the Exam Room

- Any device resembling a torture rack, even if the doctor tells you it's just a Pilates machine
- A video camera mounted on the ceiling, pointed down on you
- A Ouija board
- A swimsuit calendar (the doctor might get distracted from handling your case)
- A putting green (the doctor might get really distracted from handling your case)

Now that you've completed your recon without spotting anything too alarming, it's time to be examined!

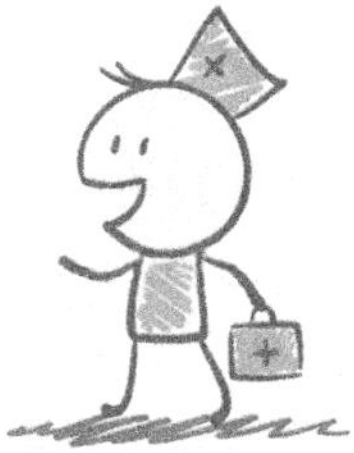

CHAPTER 3
YOUR OFFICE VISIT

I recently went to a new doctor and noticed he was located in something called "The Professional Building." I felt better right away.

—George Carlin

It's amazing how nervous people can get while waiting to see the doctor. They're hypervigilant, jumpy, and sweaty, waiting for the right moment to flee. Your office visit does not have to be that way! Let's talk about what will typically happen during your appointment so you can be prepared and cool as a cucumber.

Taking Your Vital Signs

Young doctors are taught that the reason certain things are called "vital signs" is that they are vital.

Absolutely! If you have no vital signs, your doctor's visit will be mutually unsatisfying.

Your Temperature

We take this one first, because it puts you in a different basket right off the bat. (Not literally, of course, because that would make the waiting room look freakish, though well decorated.) People often ask what number represents a fever. Many pediatricians say that if a baby has a temperature at or above 100.4, he has a fever. Some say 100.5 and up. Many docs say a fever for adults begins at 101.0; some others say at 101.5. However, we all agree that if we can fry an egg on your forehead, you've made the cut. (You're welcome—I'm glad I could clear up any confusion you may have had.)

If you do have a real fever, it politely informs us that you are sick. And as odd as this may sound, not everyone who comes to the doctor with a problem *is* actually sick. There are six broad patient categories:

1. Those who are not sick but think they are
2. Those who are not sick but wish they were
3. Those who are a little sick
4. Those who are pretty sick
5. Those who are bad sick
6. Those who have no clue they're sick (these folks are the scariest)

Fever is an objective gauge of whether or not you are sick and whether or not you should wait in the waiting room for a long time or a really long time.

Your Blood Pressure

Your blood pressure is the vital sign that will most commonly get you into trouble. A bad reading can quickly transform your routine physical from an "I'm-just-here-to-get-my-oil-changed" experience into a "Did-you-know-you-have-gasoline-leaking-out-of-your-engine-and-it-just-might-blow-up-at-any-second-unless-you-fork-over-$5000-right-now?" one!

Knowledge is power. So let's discuss what your blood pressure is and how to get the best reading possible so that you can leave the doctor's office in your own car and not in the back of a screeching ambulance.

First, a definition: Blood pressure is the measure of how much pain we medical folks can cause when we mercilessly squeeze all the blood out of a critical limb. Okay, I'm fibbing. Blood pressure is really the measure of how much *pressure* is in the blood vessels when we mercilessly squeeze all the blood out of a critical limb. This is important to know, because the more pressure you have in your vessels, the more chance they have to pop. Just kidding—you still have plenty of blood in your arm, and your vessels won't pop. It just feels like it.

A reasonable blood pressure for a grown-up is around 120/70 or under. Now, please don't get all wrapped up in whether an elevated top number or bottom number is more dangerous. The bottom line is that we want both numbers normal. How do you make them normal? Here's some official medical advice:

For twelve months before your actual doctor's appointment, I advise you to:

1. Avoid caffeine
2. Avoid alcohol
3. Avoid tobacco
4. Avoid salt
5. Avoid over-the-counter medicines
6. Avoid driving in traffic
7. Avoid arguing with your significant other
8. Avoid yelling at your children
9. Avoid thinking about your boss
10. Avoid thinking about your coworkers
11. Avoid looking at your bank account or your 401(k) balance

You get the picture. Basically, if you shut yourself up in a large plastic bubble without light, food, drink, or human interaction, you *might* have a good shot at a normal blood-pressure reading! Once again, you're welcome. Glad I could help.

Your Heart Rate

The heart rate is the Rodney Dangerfield of vital signs. It has to act super crazy in order to get any respect. The vast majority of the time, it's normal and just tags along for the ride, unnoticed and unappreciated.

Your Respiratory Rate

Believe it or not, this one doesn't even get measured routinely. If we do record it, we might eyeball it. Of course, we really shouldn't guess. But the temptation to do so is based on the fact that if you're not breathing, we should, theoretically, notice. Conversely, if you're huffing and puffing away like a freight train and all you did was walk into the room and sit down, we should, theoretically, notice that too.

Your Height and Weight

Why is it that so many people want to know their height but fly into fits of depression, anxiety, and even rage if someone suggests they step on a scale? Why do people (especially ladies) expend so much negative energy on a number?

If this is you, let me ask you: Can a number define your very being? Does your self-worth hinge upon how much you weigh? I don't know about you, but the whole sad affair makes me want to eat a donut. (On second thought, never mind—I might gain weight!)

There is a real medical reason that we doctors measure your weight. Contrary to popular opinion, we don't get a thrill out of seeing whether you've been naughty or nice in the dietary department. We look at weight when we have a bona fide need to gather data. Let's say someone comes in and says, "Doc, I feel horrible! I haven't been able to eat a thing for the last six months!" I then look at his weight. If he's lost thirty pounds, he gets a complete workup. If he's gained thirty, I suspect foul play, possibly involving donuts.

Medications and Allergies

You will be asked what medications you take and what you are allergic to. We need your full attention and complete mental clarity for this part. "I take a little red pill and a big green pill" is helpful neither to us nor to you. Why? Because even when you tell us your medications and allergies perfectly, knowledgeably, and distinctly, we can still manage to mess it up. Even when you type out a list of your medications and allergies, we can still manage to mess it up. Even when you expertly put together a thirty-minute PowerPoint presentation detailing your longstanding, nearly lethal penicillin allergy, you still, inexplicably, might manage to get penicillin. So can you just imagine what might happen if you were vague about your medications and we just guessed what they were?

Your Medical History

Once we've taken your vital signs and asked about medication, we want to find out where you currently stand, sit, or lie stricken along the continuum of bodily dysfunction. This information is critical, so it's helpful to remember to mention everything. Telling your doctor as you're walking out of the office, "Oh, *by the way,* I think I was told one time that I had a leaking aneurysm" is a surefire way to give him one.

As part of your medical history, we will obtain your family history to see how many of your family members have managed to negatively impact you genetically. This is your one chance to get your doctor to feel truly sorry for you before the next round of questioning about all of your bad personal habits.

We then delve into your "social history": If, when, and how much you drink, smoke, etc. Some folks outright lie about these things, because they sincerely want us to believe they're paragons of morality and self-control. But we can typically figure out when something is amiss, and it's really tough to shock most doctors. Honesty is always the best policy.

The Actual Visit

You're now placed in a room to await your fate, er, I mean, see the doctor or her assistant. Many folks are cared for very competently and compassionately by nurse practitioners and physician assistants. This should not cause you concern. We are all colleagues who strive to give you the best care and attention you deserve, at least until the computerized HealthPro 3000 machines take over (see Chapter 12).

Your Exam

Before your exam begins, you will likely be asked to put on a flimsy little gown. To get over this potentially humiliating hump, wear it well. Man or woman, sit tall. Cross your legs, smile, tie that little plastic belt just so. Work it! Fold a paper towel crosswise and make a little scarf for your neck. Think about how fabulous you look! This is great entertainment and reduces stress while you're waiting.

From a doctor's perspective, having the patient undress is very needful, especially in case something bad is happening. It's not uncommon to find big problems that patients simply fail to mention. "When in the world were you going to tell me about this?" I scolded, incidentally spotting an infected three-inch gaping hole in the middle of one gentleman's thigh. Denial is very much alive. Combating it with a thorough exam is a good thing.

Even if you're perfectly healthy, you may find that your exam takes a strange turn. I giggle quietly to myself when healthy people come in for their routine physicals, and I just can't seem to get it in my head that they are, in fact, healthy. I find myself interrogating these folks. "Are you absolutely, positively sure you haven't had any stomach pain, indigestion, gas, nausea, vomiting, diarrhea, or bloody stools? Do you promise to tell the truth and nothing but the truth?" I'm subconsciously on a mission to find something wrong. We doctors see so much pathology that normalcy seems bizarre. If you're healthy, forgive our odd behavior. You're a strange creature.

The EKG

EKG stands for *electrocardiogram,* or cardiogram for short. You're officially old when your doctor wants to do one on you "just in case," as if he's afraid you're going to keel over any minute. If you've never had an EKG, it's this serious little device with long ominous wires coming out of it. The nurse tells you she's going to "hook you up" to it. Your first thought is to bolt, half-naked, out of there, because electrocution was not on your list of things to do today. But you've seen something similar to this on TV, and no one got electrocuted. Then again, maybe they did, and you missed it because you left the living room to get a snack.

The good news is that the EKG is painless; it just gently records the electricity produced by your heart. How neat is that? Did you know that you're a human power plant? Yes, you! The bad news is that sometimes we have to *do things* in order to get a readable tracing (creepy music here). I'll spare you the details, but the hairy guys know what I'm talking about. If you see an otherwise hairy man in a gown wandering aimlessly around the parking lot with patches of chest hair missing, looking like he lost a fight with a weasel, don't think ill of him. He's just had an EKG and needs time to recover.

Shots

Before you leave the exam room, your doctor will earnestly insist that you have some sort of shot. Have you ever wondered why shots are such a big deal to medical folks? Of course we want to protect you from tetanus. But the real reason goes deeper: Surgeon envy. Many internists secretly have this. Internists are inescapably more like Clark Kent than Superman. Many of us take great care of sick folks in the hospital and do office procedures to alleviate distress and diagnose problems, but it's not the same as getting our hands inside the body, taking disease between our fingers, and wrangling it into submission. When I give someone a shot as an internist, it's my chance to do something tangible to stave off a horrific, high-stakes disease or two and be a real heroine. In the scope of my practice, I can't swoop down and remove somebody's gangrenous gallbladder. I mean I *could,* but the guy most likely wouldn't be fixed. I mean, he'd be *fixed* all right, but not "fixed" fixed. That's why doctors love to give shots.

Blood Work

We've now reached the pinnacle of your physical exam experience—getting stuck for lab tests. On the one hand, you're curious to find out how your insides are doing. Is your cholesterol okay? Are you anemic? Are you still managing to evade the specter of diabetes that has plagued your family for generations?

On the other hand, you hate the thought of playing pincushion. You think, "Can't they come up with something that doesn't hurt? Technology has sent folks to the moon, enabled them to live in zero gravity for months, and created satellites, robot-assisted surgery, and virtual reality. Why can't science fix this one little thing?"

I hear you, 100 percent. I hate getting blood work done too. But experienced phlebotomists will typically get your blood on the first or second try. If not, they'll be wise enough to leave you alone and try again another day. If you happen to get some well-meaning but misguided person who has no qualms about doing stick number four, five, six, or beyond, run.

Sticker Shock

Let's be honest. You're anxious about how much this whole visit is going to cost. You pray that whatever blood work your doctor orders won't cost you an arm and a leg. You're also hoping she won't order expensive tests that your insurance company—if you have one—won't cover. You want an X-ray, but only a really cheap one that tells her all she needs to know.

Alas, it's not that simple. Our doctor brains operate in figure-it-out mode. You come in with a problem, and our job is to figure it out. We want to figure it out. We're trained to figure it out. We feel really good about ourselves if we figure it out. We wish we could just talk to you, examine you, and then diagnose your problem with complete and total certainty. But sometimes we can't, and we dislike being uncertain.

It's perfectly legal to talk to your doctor before she starts spending all of your money. It's also perfectly legal for her to accommodate your request for fiscal restraint, or as typically occurs, to convince you otherwise:

Dr. Jones: "Well, Mr. Smith, I've examined you from head to toe, and I think your bad headaches are probably just from severe tension. But I'd like you to get an MRI of your brain just in case."

Mr. Smith: "How much will that cost?"

Dr. Jones (clueless, making something up): "Uh—about $1000 or so" (unbeknownst to Dr. Jones, it may cost more, *way* more), "but it depends on your insurance." (Good save—she's hoping her referral coordinator will be able to give Mr. Smith a more accurate number. She went to school to be a doctor, not a biller.)

Mr. Smith (severe headache returning): "I just can't afford it, Doc. What else can you do?"

Dr. Jones: "I could put on a mask and chant and throw chicken bones in your direction. If the bones point toward you in a certain way, you might live."

Mr. Smith: "So you really think I need an MRI?"

Dr. Jones: "It's the right thing to do. And I don't want to be a bad doctor. I want you to have the best care possible." (Translation: "I don't want to get sued if I miss something. I have two kids in college.")

Am I saying the only reason doctors order tests is that they don't want to be sued? Of course not! It's one of the three main reasons they order tests:

Reason #1: To find out if their initial diagnostic impression is right. We *love* being right! Oh yes, and to take care of you.

Reason #2: To not get sued.

Reason #3: Did I mention to not get sued?

You may be thinking, "How is it even possible that a doctor has no idea about how much a test or procedure costs?" That is an excellent question. The answer: Price is a SECRET. Even to us doctors.

Let's say I'm caring for Grandma. Grandma lives on a fixed income. If I knew what different medical facilities in my area were charging for Test X, I would, in good faith, steer Grandma to the cheapest facility, even if it were in a different (read competing) hospital system. This, I believe, is one of the biggest reasons for price secrecy.

And even if all the area facilities made their prices available, this knowledge would be incomplete, because the amount that Grandma's insurance will pick up is a secret too. Also, prices secretly vary by geographical area and target market.

Whenever I get proactive and try to find out how much Test X is going to cost Grandma, it's nigh unto impossible to get a real figure. Since apparently the Medical Test Price Police are bugging the phones, I can lose hours of time making multiple dead-end phone calls to people who are unable or unwilling to divulge the data.

So the best I can say is, "Well, Grandma, it looks like your test will cost about $500. Or $1500. Or more. I have no idea." How reprehensible, when Grandma already has to make the tough decision whether or not to buy crackers with her cat food this month. When people go to the grocery store, the prices of items are clearly marked. The 99-cent loaf of bread is next to the $2.99 bread, and shoppers can easily decide which one fits their particular lifestyle and budget. Our medical system will not begin to improve until there is price transparency. Until that time, doctors are stuck guessing how much tests cost.

The only times I've been privy to costs of tests is from the feedback of (1) irate patients, (2) irate family members, and (3) myself, after having more tests as I've gotten older. Until the public outcry over lack of price transparency gets loud enough, you'll continue to be in the dark too.

At least your doctor means well. Doesn't that make you feel better?

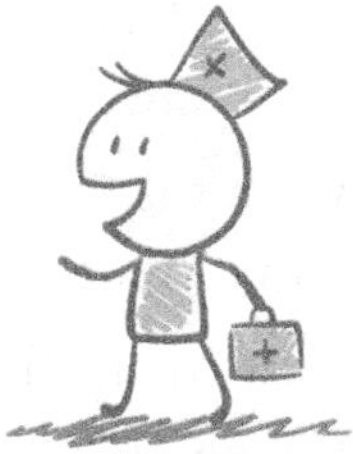

CHAPTER 4
THE EMERGENCY ROOM

Isn't it a bit unnerving that doctors call what they do "Practice?"
—George Carlin

TYPICALLY A MAJOR bodily malfunction occurs in the middle of the night, when you're most scared, helpless, and alone. Chest pain, shortness of breath, severe headache, and injury certainly qualify among many other reasons to go to the ER. If you're not sure, just go.

Certain people who visit the ER, however, are not truly ill. They routinely use the ER as a doctor's office, requesting refills of Viagra, paternity tests, and notes to stay home from work. This behavior clogs up the ER and makes it hard for you to be cared for quickly when you're urgently sick. (If you can't afford a doctor, get help in Chapter 11.)

"But Dr. Woodhouse," you may ask, "isn't that what the triage nurse in the ER is for?" (*Triage* comes from the French, meaning *to sort.*) Yes, but she's *tired* (from the English, meaning *too through*). The people who are not acutely ill are wearing her out, especially when they keep coming up to her every five minutes asking how much longer the wait will be. So to preserve her sanity, she ratchets down her triage criteria to "those who are actively bleeding on the floor."

As a spouse or concerned significant other, you may have the opposite problem. Your loved one is seriously ill, but refuses to go to the ER. You've been struggling with this loved one all day, and now it's 3 a.m. He's becoming less loveable by the minute. You're exhausted, stressed, and at your wits' end. You have my permission, as a trained medical professional, to knock him out with a brick and drag his limp body to the car. The ER doctor will sort it all out when you get there. I'm using the personal pronoun "he" quite intentionally. Fellas, just go and take care of the problem, as you would if it were a problem with your car. Save your ladylove the extra pain and heartache.

The Waiting Room

First of all, the initials ER do not simply stand for emergency room, but also for "everybody retch", from the Latin *E Pluribus Retchitus,* which is a major ongoing activity in emergency rooms. The other major activity is looking around wistfully in pain and misery waiting to be seen. Bound by human suffering and the effects of time, the folks in the ER waiting room become a feral tribe, not unlike those featured on reality TV shows. An obviously injured man on crutches assists a frail, elderly woman slumped in a wheelchair. A disheveled man is wedged in a corner mumbling that the CIA is reading his thoughts. A sick but selfless woman looks after everybody, wheeling and dealing, doing PR for other patients at the nurses' station. Apathetic moms are impervious to the piercing screams of their feverish infants, and frustrated people are talking much too loudly on their cell phones. It's quite a raucous scene, and it's quite challenging to wait there for five, six, or ten hours, or until your toddler calls and asks for money to go to college.

I'm ashamed to admit that once (years ago, when I was a young doctor and full of hope), I sent a sick, uninsured patient from the clinic to a major metropolitan ER with explicit instructions, right before he walked in the ER door, to put several

Alka-Seltzer tablets into his mouth to make it look like he was foaming. I reasoned that he'd get past the triage nurse quickly and into the back sooner. But I was wrong. In my defense, he probably didn't do it right. He likely came across as a pathetic, desperate patient trying to access care. Which he was, but it wasn't supposed to look so obvious.

When you're finally called to go to a room, you'll feel like you've achieved a major victory. And the sum total of the group's dreams and aspirations will be carried by you into the unknown.

The ER Experience

Long, cold, noisy, and uncomfortable. And that's just the trip back to your room. Exactly what happens next depends on your individual situation, but be sure it involves a lot more waiting. Waiting to be seen by the nurse. Waiting to be seen by the tech. Waiting to be seen by the housekeeper, who always seems to have an intense, immediate need to empty the trashcan in your room during your most intimate (i.e., unclothed) moments. Waiting to be seen by the medical student. Waiting to be seen by the resident. By the time you get to meet the one human being who is ultimately responsible for your care, the ER attending physician, you've forgotten everything, including your name.

This is the medical establishment's way of making you look like an oafish patient who can't be counted on to keep the bed warm, let alone provide a thoughtful, tangible history they can work with. Sample chart entry: "Patient cannot recall what brought him here—will discharge after vigorous soap-suds enema times four." This is the same technique used by countless customer-service call centers. There's only so long you can stay on hold listening to elevator music. When an operator finally picks up your call, you're a mindless lump of drool with no clue why you called in the first place. It's incredibly effective.

Once your ER workup is complete, the housekeeper will give you your discharge paperwork. Your paper will say something helpful like "CHEST PAIN, NONCARDIAC—GET LOST." Make sure you bring this paper back to your doctor, preferably without grease spots, blood, or phlegm on it. She will need this paper to guess what kind of workup you might have had in the ER. She will accomplish this by holding the paper up against her forehead and saying, "Ommm," thereby completing the loop and ensuring your medical problem has been thoroughly evaluated from all angles. Until electronic medical records are the norm and are shared amongst different (read competing) hospital systems, we doctors will continue to rely on ESP when you return for your follow-up visit.

But what if you're admitted from the ER into the hospital? Don't worry. Unless you have a clear-cut, slam-dunk problem like not breathing, odds are you and your loved ones will be the last to know. Deciding to admit a patient is an intricate, multifaceted decision that takes into account your current stability, your potential for getting worse, and your ability to pay the bill. (Just joking! Really!)

Doctors often hem and haw about borderline admissions, and it's fascinating to watch the ER and on-call physicians of the various specialties politely discussing whether you should stay in the hospital or be discharged with close outpatient follow-up. Each doctor has his or her own opinion, which the other colleague will respectfully point out is wrong. Sometimes the discussions become more spirited, and the "yo mama" cracks start to fly.

So this process takes time. And just when you think you are going be discharged and see the light of day, you're informed quietly by a shadowy figure in a trench coat that one guy amidst the gaggle of doctors has had a random thought that you should stay in the hospital, just in case. You dismiss it because the ER attending physician hasn't personally informed you of this herself. You visually scan the room for signs of your underwear, which were unceremoniously dumped in a brown paper bag during your evaluation, and wait to be unhooked from the IV and monitor. Instead, hands from out of nowhere kidnap you and rush your bed, Mob-style, into a rickety service elevator, with no witnesses. You've just been admitted.

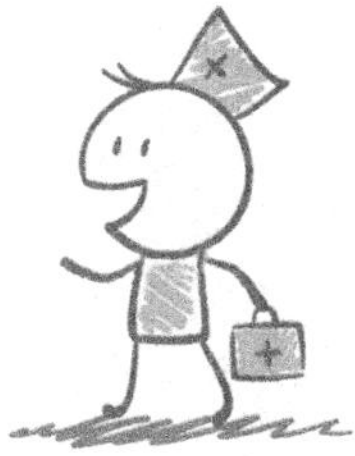

CHAPTER 5

YOUR HOSPITAL STAY

A hospital bed is like a parked taxi with the meter running.

—Groucho Marx

NOT ALL HOSPITAL STAYS are created equal. Your experience will vary greatly depending on where you're placed.

The Intensive Care Unit

If you wind up in the ICU (medical, surgical, cardiac, etc.), this chapter isn't for you. You are seriously ill, and possibly unconscious, making reading this book very difficult. Also, your sense of humor is likely to be impaired. Focus your energies on getting better and getting transferred to the step-down unit.

The Step-Down Unit

Step-down units house patients who are either coming out of intensive care or might have to go into it—folks who need close monitoring because they could go either way. You can spot them by those handsome little heart monitors they wear on their chests. A heart monitor is a special badge, a prominent emblem indicating that someone is really concerned for you and your well-being. The unmonitored patients look at you jealously, green with envy. That is, until your monitor goes off; then they're not the only ones looking green.

Outside of the occasional personal emergency, being in step-down is not that exciting. You know you have truly arrived and experienced the American medical system at its best when you get admitted to the internal medicine floor.

On the Floor (Not Literally)

The "Floor"—where nonsurgical, non-critically-ill patients are cared for—is one of the most colorful places *not* to sleep in the hospital. Every doctor-to-be does at least one inpatient adult medicine Floor rotation during his or her third year of medical school. This rotation is the reason many medical students change their minds and decide to go to law school instead.

The Floor is truly hard to describe. Fighting illness in the hospital is like being in a war. Our mission is to get you better and out of there, but the medical problem—the enemy—typically doesn't go down easily. Tension and struggle, bad days and less bad days are the norm. Everyone's a combatant. Patients are fighting to get better, the doctors are fighting to make them better, and the staff is fighting to get their jobs done. Picture shell-shocked ill people wandering around, noise, confusion, and bad food, and you're on the right track.

I confess I've never trained in or worked on a hospital Floor that didn't have the distinctive odor of hard combat. So my viewpoint may be skewed. "My dear Dr. Woodhouse," one of my more privileged colleagues may drawl, "when I work at Heavenly Saint Ignatious Perfectus Mercy Grace Hospital, eunuchs carry me around in a chaise and feed me peeled grapes." And some of you readers with excellent insurance may have had a hospital stay akin to being in a plush five-star luxury hotel. Fantastic! I'm glad you're reading this so you're prepared for reality when your insurance changes.

Being an Inpatient

As a hospitalized patient, you have a myriad of unique challenges that you must successfully surmount, including:

Your illness itself. It's truly unpleasant to be sick and in pain.

Your confinement. You're trapped. You can't go home. You're too tired and weak to even think about calling a cab. Some people do try, but typically that turns out badly.

Your very own doctors and nurses. We constantly interrupt your sleep. We poke holes in you with needles at every opportunity. We ask you the same dumb questions over and over. We touch you everywhere with really cold hands that you're not sure we've even washed. And more often than not, we get irritated when you need something.

Noise. Your apparently deaf neighbor in the next bed has his TV blaring. Amazingly, he's not only fast asleep but snoring. Loudly. Overhead pages for nurses and doctors and everyone else in the whole hospital are incessant. Your IV line is beeping nonstop; either your medicine infusion is complete, or something has gone horribly wrong. Even if you have a private room and the door is closed, a medical team has managed to find their way to right outside your door, talking and laughing loudly as if they were at home (we are; we spend all our lives at work. We sometimes forget you're trying to rest—sorry).

Anxious thoughts. Will you get to leave the hospital before your life savings is gone? Is someone stealing your mail? Are your pets all right? Did you remember to turn down the thermostat? That horrible hacking cough of your neighbor's couldn't possibly be contagious, otherwise they wouldn't have put him in here with you, right? Right?

Environmental issues. Your room is either icy cold or boiling hot. Your bed feels like it's made out of a slab of rock, à la *The Flintstones.* And somehow the nurse call bell is always way underneath the bed, completely out of reach.

The food. I know. Some hospitals do have downright nasty food. But the vast majority of hospitals have gotten better over the years. The main problem now is that hospital food is healthier than what most Americans eat every day. That's why it doesn't taste right and there never seems to be enough of it. If you have high blood pressure, you will get a low-salt tray. If you have diabetes, you will get a low-sugar tray. If you have high blood pressure *and* diabetes, you will have issues. My grandmother was in this last group and simply refused to eat because the hospital food wasn't tasty (i.e., fat-infested) enough. By essentially going on a hunger strike, she forced the family to sneak out and get her fast food. Do you know how difficult it is to cover up the smell of a hot greasy burger and fries in a hospital ward?

Random thoughts. You find your mind wandering. "Did someone die in this bed? What about in this gown I have on? Where's my wallet? My glasses? I need to update my will. I'm stopping smoking. I'm losing fifty pounds as soon as I get out of here." And so on.

Visitors who refuse to go home. It's wonderful that people bring you balloons, flowers, and cards. And on a practical level, this alerts the hospital staff, "Yes, I do have plenty of friends and family who are watching and care about how this hospital stay works out, if you know what I mean." It's fantastic that your visitors pray for you, comfort you, and remind you of all the good things waiting for you when you leave the hospital. But some folks can't perceive when it's time for them to go home. You get tired. Sometimes you just want to be left alone. And sometimes you know their only intention is to gossip about you when they leave.

INPATIENT Q&A:

Q: *I feel weak and tired all of the time. Why doesn't my doctor just admit me into the hospital and run a bunch of tests on me there?*

A: It used to be that we docs could send folks to the hospital for a tune-up. Those days are over. Now we have to supply the powers-that-be with a quantifiable, black-and-white *reason* to put you in the hospital, like "patient is not breathing." You have to be half-dead both to get into and to remain in the hospital. If by God's grace you start inching away from the precipice of death, somebody from the insurance mafia is sure to leave your doctor threatening entries in your chart: "Get Mr. Smith out NOW, OR ELSE." What's the "or else"? Your doctor may suffer physical violence, *and* your hospital bill may not be fully paid. Also, no longer are you discharged from the hospital when you're all better. These days, you get discharged as soon as you can be sick at home. Hope that helps.

Q: *I've been in the hospital all week, and now it's the weekend. Who are all these new people taking care of me?*

A: Depending on your hospital, the team of doctors and nurses you see on the weekend may be completely different from the one that normally cares for you Monday through Friday. Hopefully, information about you has been transferred completely and accurately; don't be afraid to speak up if things don't seem to be moving in the right direction. Also, very few nonemergency tests get done on the weekend. Assuming your body cooperates, the weekend may be a good time to catch up on some much-needed sleep. Unfortunately, the weekend is also the time when all of the folks who never called you or gave you a passing thought for years will show up uninvited when you least feel like seeing them.

Q: *I'm so glad you brought that up, Dr. Woodhouse! I have unwanted family members or other people in my room who just aren't getting the message that I'm really tired and they need to go home already. What should I do?*

A: This is a common problem for many hospitalized patients. It's also a common problem for anyone who ever has guests in her home. Unfortunately, the usual fixes—like yawning loudly and exclaiming, "Look at the time! I didn't know it was so late!" or refilling their glasses up only halfway—may not work in the hospital setting. Your visitors may be so determined to give you emotional support by any means necessary that they will never leave. Simply being honest with them and asking them politely to exit stage right might hurt their feelings. You'd like the decision for them to leave to be completely theirs. But there *is* something you can do: You can use your current illness to your advantage.

For starters, cough violently and frequently in their general direction. It's even better if you manage to cough up some blood for extra emphasis. You could also ask your visitors to hand you your bedpan. You might mention that you don't know when you'll no longer be contagious, or abruptly call the nurse to give you fresh bed linens ASAP. Your unwanted visitors will get the drift. Otherwise you'll simply have to call Security.

Q: *What are medical "rounds"?*

A: Rounds are an important, time-honored medical tradition in teaching hospitals. The medical team walks from one patient room to another throughout the day to make sure you are still alive. The intern sees you first, typically at the crack of dawn; next, the upper-year resident will come around and examine you.

Provided that you *are* in fact still alive, the head of your treatment team, the attending physician, will formally round on you with the entire team later on that morning, well after she has secured her coffee and donut. A whole crowd of about ten white-coated folks will suddenly barge into your room unannounced, typically right when you're in the middle of eating breakfast. With the whole team watching, the attending physician will first banter genially with you and then start poking at you to show the team an interesting "finding," i.e., something your body does or has that is not normal.

The young doctors-in-training are supposed to burn these "findings" forever into their memories and use them to diagnose illnesses in other sick people in the future without the help of CT scans or MRIs. Really.

Q: *What is "pimping"?*

A: Pimping is unfortunately another time-honored tradition in medical training, but you as a patient will likely never witness it. Attending physicians and upper-year residents are careful to completely embarrass their medical students and interns out in the hallway, where only their fellow classmates, nurses, and random passersby can witness their gross ignorance. Historically, the intention was to educate young doctors via the Socratic method, whereby each student is asked increasingly difficult questions until they're nonplussed and in tears. The interrogator wields all the control and power during this exchange, and an insensitive instructor can fracture a student's fledgling confidence. When that student goes home later that night to study, he studies less to obtain knowledge and help his fellow man than he does in order not to be embarrassed in front of everyone that badly again.

Q: *I am sick and tired of being in this rock-hard hospital bed. I'm not feeling as lousy as I was when I got here, and nobody's telling me anything. Can't I just leave?*

A: It's tempting to leave the hospital before you're officially dismissed, especially if you start to feel a little better. The problem with leaving the hospital Against Medical Advice (AMA) is that you might "bounce back," meaning that you run the risk of being hospitalized all over again. But if a sane, non-suicidal patient wants to sign himself out, we doctors can't prevent him.

Increasingly, people sign out early because they simply can't afford to stay in the hospital any longer. Others are single moms who worry about their children. If you're considering leaving

> AMA, please use sound judgment. Is it more economical to get better and stay that way, or to leave early, feel marginal, and have to come back in? Sometimes a day or two can make a big difference.

Having Surgery in the Hospital

Generally, internists and surgeons avoid each other like the plague. Why? One theory is that many internists secretly believe they're smarter, while many surgeons secretly believe they're more effective. Internists are jealous because surgeons are palpably curing disease, and surgeons are likewise jealous because internists have more opportunity to go home during daylight hours. This unspoken rivalry causes us to stay out of each other's way, which works well until a patient starts to get really sick.

When a patient is hospitalized, sometimes medication is the way to go. Sometimes it's cold, hard steel. Other times it's both. Neither specialty has the corner on the "make it better" market. It's a beautiful thing when a surgeon swoops down and snatches up an internist's patient with a perforated intestine. A surgeon likely feels the same way when an internist deftly handles whatever chronic, nonsurgical medical problem the surgeon doesn't have the emotional energy to deal with. The bottom line is that we need each other. And as a patient, you need us to play nice together. This is how the general experience might go.

Scenario One: Your Surgery is Unplanned (Emergency):

1. You have a life-threatening illness; you're unconscious, or nearly so.
2. A hazy blob of a person in a white coat (you highly doubt it's an angel) tells you in a faraway voice that you need surgery right now, or else.
3. You, or more likely, your loved ones, agree to the surgery because the general consensus is that you need to keep on being alive.

Scenario Two: Your Surgery is Planned

1. You hem and haw for months about whether or not to have surgery at all. You solicit opinions from everybody, including perfect strangers in the supermarket checkout line. Truth be told, you don't totally trust your doctor to be completely honest with you.
2. You wonder if you'll still have a job when you get back from your surgery.

3. You decide to get a second opinion, because the first surgeon you consulted had Band-Aids on his fingers. When you meet the other doctor for the second opinion, you discover that he's in the middle of a painful divorce and doesn't appear to have the will to live. Return to Step 1.

4. When you finally find a surgeon who seems both proficient and mentally sound, you decide to go for it because the pain/discomfort/danger/social embarrassment of your particular medical condition is unbearable. And just in case something should happen on the operating table, you tell your family that you love them and not to blow all of the insurance money on movies and pizza.

Let's assume you have your surgery and everything goes smoothly in the operating room. What can you expect next?

1. You wake up in pain, barely able to perceive a plastic bag full of urine that's unceremoniously draped across your bed rail. "Whose is that?" you inquire irritably, before you realize, even more irritably, that it's yours.

2. You take a pain pill and fall into fitful, restless pseudo-sleep while various family

members and friends attempt to engage you in fruitless conversation.

3. Days go by like this, barring a setback, complication, or therapeutic misadventure.

Notice I'm bringing up the issue of complications when you're an inpatient on the surgical side of the hospital, and not when you're on the internal medicine side. How interesting. Anyway, let's discuss the differences between these important occurrences so that you'll be able to recognize them.

A *setback* is what happens when you find your wallet has been stolen out of the dresser next to your hospital bed. In one of your medication-induced hazes, you loudly exclaim your intentions for the thief as soon as you can get out of bed. And voilà, your wallet is mysteriously "set back." This is an extremely rare phenomenon.

A *complication* is when an anticipated result, such as you getting better, does not exactly work out as planned. This is something unforeseen, which is no one's fault per se. For example, you're given a lifesaving antibiotic that you just happen to be seriously allergic to.

A *therapeutic misadventure* is when everything goes wrong, triggered by an unfortunate decision or two (or three) somewhere along the chain of care. It's akin to dominoes falling; where you end up is miles away from where you started. Hospitals earnestly try to avoid these by designing processes and systems to keep you safe. And we doctors are ethically, morally, and legally bound to inform you if you're in the midst of such a misadventure. Does that help? No? At least it has an official name.

Who is most at risk for these phenomena? This is an important question; after all, it would be great if you knew ahead of time that you were wearing a bull's-eye. Surprisingly, medical professionals seem to have the highest risk of heinous happenstance. For some inexplicable reason, nurses are especially prone. If a patient tells me she's a nurse, I've got the night-vision goggles out, constantly vigilant for weird things to happen.

Back to your inpatient surgery stay:

4. Your crowning moment is to make it to the bedside commode unassisted, with Herculean effort.

5. You're informed that you will need to get out, I mean, be discharged, early tomorrow morning even though you haven't officially walked yet nor eaten solid food. This is at the insistent prodding of your insurance company, which is already peeved that you made it into the hospital in the first place.

6. You point this out to your nurse, who pluckily encourages you to get out of bed and practice laps around the ward in preparation for an independent life at home. Privately, she sighs deeply, knowing that her hands are tied.

7. You point this out to the intern, the resident, and the attending surgeon, who all encourage you to get out of bed and practice laps, but who likewise sigh deeply, knowing that their hands are tied.

8. When morning comes, you console yourself with the thought that at least you can recuperate in your own home and in your own bed, and slowly shuffle down the hall into your waiting car.

A Who's Who Guide to Your Inpatient Team

When you're in the emergency room, it's not too critical to get to know who is taking care of you. Why? Because you're either in or out when you're in the ER—"in" in the sense that you're really sick and there's no way you're leaving (except when an unscrupulous hospital finds out you're uninsured and dumps you out on the street) or "out" in the sense that you're dischargeable, meaning the ER doctors are betting you'll probably make it back alive to your primary care doctor's office for follow-up in the next forty-eight to seventy-two hours. The vast majority of people are, thankfully, in the latter category. Therefore, the pace of ER patient flow is fairly brisk, with little time for deep relationships to form between patient and physician. Most ER doctors prefer it that way.

On the inpatient side of the hospital, however, things are different. The focus shifts from quickly assessing your condition to letting medical students, subinterns, interns, and residents all take a crack at you. (If you are unfortunate enough not to be admitted to a teaching hospital, you're missing out on a wonderful, time-honored medical tradition. You're missing out on a wonderful opportunity to play a vital role in the education of the doctors of tomorrow. You're missing out on a wonderful opportunity to have up to four examinations every single day!)

Here's a guide to key players on your inpatient team. After all, you should be prepared when you're finally able to get some sleep and a noisy gaggle of eight strangers suddenly barges in and starts demanding things of you: "Sit up," "Breathe deeply," "Roll over," "Show us that tattoo we've heard about," etc.

The Nurses

The inpatient staff includes not only the nurses, but also nursing assistants, receptionists, administrators, and a whole host of other people who just drop by (chaplains, educators, social workers, therapists, and random lost folks who wander into your room by mistake). But by far, you'll have the most intimate contact with your nurses. So it's critical to understand the milieu in which most inpatient nurses work.

In these powerfully heady days of cost containment, nurses across the country are being asked to care for more and more patients with less and less help. Your nurses may very well be stretched very thinly. Crazy coworkers make things worse. The life-and-death struggles inherent in hospital medicine are stressful enough. But if you throw in an abusive, tantrum-throwing attending physician on top of a twenty-plus patient caseload, you might just end up with a slightly crabby nurse.

Try hard to develop pleasant relationships with your nurses. They are your real caregivers while you're in the hospital. Wise doctors can testify to this. When a physician needs something handled, a good nurse can get it D-O-N-E. It's an excellent thing when your nurses find you easy to deal with. One suggestion: Try not to holler. Yelling "Nurse! Nurse!" all day long instead of using the call bell is not conducive to a friendly relationship with your nurse.

In the old days, hospital nurses would spend the better part of the day chasing down the doctors to clarify hastily scrawled orders. Now, thanks to electronic medical records, nurses spend the better part of the day chasing down the doctors to clarify hastily entered computer orders. The nurses attempt to do this with phones or pagers, to which most doctors have become completely deaf. This forces the nurses to call the doctors repeatedly. So if you've asked your nurse for some Tylenol and it seems inordinately slow in coming, it's because she's glued to the phone waiting for the doctor's call back. Now you know.

The Doctors

If you are admitted to a *nonteaching* hospital, only the physicians directly responsible for your care will be touching you. But if you're a patient in a *teaching* hospital, you have your very own team. I wish I could say that you're the coach, or the manager, but actually, you're the ball. Sorry!

If you're admitted to the hospital through the emergency room, you may meet two members of your team before you get assigned a hospital room: the medical student/subintern and your intern. Next, the resident will come by and grunt at you, ensuring that none of these people are planning things that might inadvertently kill you. If you're admitted in the evening, you won't see the head attending physician until the next day. She's at home busily thanking God that she has residents to help her out.

The Medical Students

These bright and eager young people are college graduates who have surmounted the hugely competitive process of getting into and staying in medical school. Most are in traditional four-year training programs, so they've spent the last two years studying the human body in great detail using books and cadavers. Now they get the chance to handle real live human beings, and ones who happen to be sick at that. This is a *major* deal.

You can recognize medical students by their short white coats. Generally speaking, the length and detail of a doctor's lab coat denotes her status in the medical hierarchy. Medical students are typically smiling, flush with fresh optimism and hope for the future, at least for the first few months. Their mission is to learn how to perform an accurate medical history and physical exam (on you) and begin to learn to diagnose and treat (you). That means you'll be seeing them *a lot.*

The good news is that they've only been assigned a few patients. That makes them the only people on the doctor team who have the time to truly listen to you. Also, some of them still like the idea of helping sick people. The bad news is that technically, they're not doctors yet. They should always introduce themselves as students, and if they don't, you should politely ask them who they are. As much as you're able (given the fact that you're sick), be gracious and let them spend time with you. Let them fumble as they learn to examine you (within reason). You might be helping train the world's most famous doctor! Most of us doctors will never forget our first patients in medical school.

The Subinterns ("Sub-I's")

Subinterns are fourth-year medical students who are about to graduate from medical school. They wear short coats like their third-year fellows, but their confidence is soaring. Instead of bright-eyed wonder, they exude an air of self-assured boldness.

Their mission is to practice being interns by actively advancing diagnoses and treatment plans on your case, all under the watchful eye of the supervising resident or intern. They are to develop a sense of competence until the intern year hits.

Give them encouragement and tell them what fantastic doctors they'll be. They'll need every ounce of strength they can muster for their upcoming internships.

The Interns

Ah, the illustrious, celebrated interns. The media has made interns the most famous doctors in training, romanticizing their naïveté in the face of incredible life-and-death responsibilities. They're still human because they've not yet fully transitioned into full doctorhood, so people relate to them more readily.

What are interns? Interns are "real" doctors in that they have graduated from medical school and can legally put an MD behind their names. They're in their first year of residency in whatever discipline they have chosen, be it family practice, internal medicine, etc. Technically, interns are residents. But because the first year of residency training is so special, they get their very own designation. And one quick clarification: Internists (doctors who practice internal medicine, which is the care of the adult patient) are not interns. I can't count the number of times I've introduced myself as an internist and had patients sweetly inquire how I like being an intern.

Interns have training licenses and can't function independently yet. However, their learning curve is fast and steep. Squeaky new interns in July morph, like butterflies, into sleek, efficient, and experienced professionals by June of the following year. It is an amazing transformation.

Interns may be harder to recognize because their appearance depends on the time of year you see them. If you catch them in July when they're newly minted, their chests will poke out proudly from their new long white coats. By November, they carry about an exhausted, defeated cast, and they are wrinkled and smelly from not having had any time or energy to bathe anytime in the near past. By June they are steely hard, highly competent, and anxious to move up the occupational food chain.

Their mission? In a word, everything. They are the workhorses for your case. They assist in developing your treatment plan, but they're also the ones who make the plan happen. No task is too lowly, too menial, too obscure, or too far-fetched for the humble intern. Go easy on your intern. Smile at him from time to time if you're able, and tell him it's going to be all right.

The Upper-Year Residents

Upper-year residents have successfully completed their internship year and are now completing additional years of training. A number of residencies are three years long, so the upper-years are second- and third-year residents who are nearing the end of their training and are functioning independently.

In general, second-year residents directly supervise the interns and manage "teams" of patients, which may be twenty to thirty patients deep or more. Third-year residents supervise all the team members and all the patients. Upper-year residents also provide consultation for other medical disciplines, teach the interns how to perform invasive procedures, and "run codes," i.e., resuscitate patients whose hearts have stopped beating or who are not breathing. As you can imagine, they are extremely busy people. You can easily recognize them because they carry more phones and beepers than seems humanly possible.

The upper-years' primary mission is to make sure the interns don't kill you, especially in July. They are focused on finishing residency so that they can have a less brutal call schedule and finally get some sleep. They are smart, dedicated, capable, hardworking, efficient, and ever-vigilant to see that things are going smoothly for you during your hospital stay. Ask them lots of questions. They enjoy being able to showcase their knowledge and expertise.

The Attending Physicians

Attending physicians are the full-fledged docs who have completed their residencies. They can be brand spanking new or have been practicing forever. They're the ones who teach and supervise the whole medical team and who are legally responsible for your care while you're in the hospital. Their lab coats are long, white, sleek, and actually starched. Their shoes are shined, and they tend to dress much, much better than everyone else. In a teaching hospital, this means they do much less of the real work.

Attendings ensure that the treatment plan proposed by the team is reasonable, efficient, and, dare I add, cost-effective. They do their best not to get themselves or the hospital sued. They attempt to train up a generation of sharp young doctors so that when they themselves get old and feeble, they'll have somebody halfway competent to care for them. And they endeavor to do all of this before 5 p.m. if at all possible.

Staying Halfway Sane in the Hospital

Remember that for the overwhelming majority of folks on the medical floor, the stay is only temporary. Odds are fairly good you'll make it home.

Don't be afraid to nicely ask for what you need. If you need a more comfortable mattress, ask. If you need the heat turned up in your room because your IV tubing is frozen, ask. If you need the staff to talk more quietly outside your room, ask. If you need to sweetly and politely draw the curtain between you and your seemingly tuberculous neighbor, feel free.

And while you're waiting to get better, this is an excellent time to talk to God. Honestly, laid out on a hospital bed, what else are you going to do? When else are you going to be so in touch with your humanity and with the brevity of life? And what else can possibly do you as much good as asking for and receiving divine help? If you truly reach out to Him, the great news is that He will show up. You lose nothing by trying, and you have everything to gain. See the Epilogue for more details.

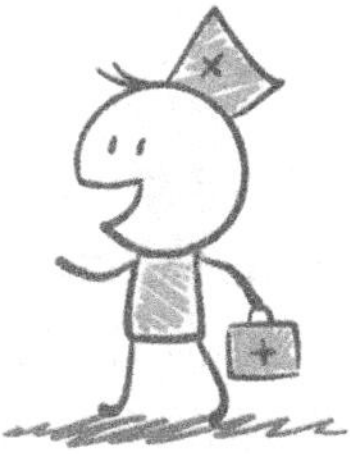

CHAPTER 6
PROPER PATIENT ETIQUETTE

Joy, temperance, and repose slam the door
on the doctor's nose.

—Henry Wadsworth Longfellow

YOU'VE MADE IT THROUGH your office visit, the ER, and the hospital—fantastic! But medical care is a two-way street. Let's discuss proper techniques for being a good patient so that your relationship with your physician can operate at its most mutually satisfying level.

What's the easiest way to be a good patient? To not be a bad one.

How Not to Be a Bad Patient

I personally feel that I have no business writing this section. But several doctor friends gently persuaded me (at gunpoint) to submit this highly relevant and critical topic for your review. Outside of a patient's mishandling a narcotic prescription (forging it, sharing it, selling it, "losing" it, and especially lying about it), one of the biggest things that can make someone a bad patient is noncompliance.

These days, doctors are being encouraged to use the more benevolent term "nonadherence" to include patients who desire to heed medical advice, but are hindered by external factors beyond their control. For instance, some people get laid off and are simply unable to afford their medication. But I'm not talking about nonadherence. I'm talking about old-fashioned noncompliance, the willful disdain of a highly recommended course of action despite the obvious danger of bodily harm.

> Noncompliance:
> (n.), Old Eng.; "non," *without* + "compliance,"
> *a clue that you are not the doctor.*

I'm a noncompliant patient. There—I said it. The last time I was given an antibiotic prescription following a dental procedure, my attitude was, "I don't need this garbage." And it got worse. "I'll just save it for if I get really sick," I thought, as if my dentist didn't know what he was doing. And I fuss at my patients for not taking their medications correctly!

What is it about the human psyche that makes people want to be always in control and free to make unwise decisions? I'm not talking about having a side effect from a medication and discontinuing it—that's legitimate. I'm talking about when folks go to a doctor for advice, refuse to heed the advice, and then come back for more advice. This is what hardcore noncompliance looks like:

Dr. James (during a two-month follow-up visit for high cholesterol): "Hello, Mr. Smith! How are you doing on the new cholesterol pill?"

Mr. Smith (affably): "What cholesterol pill?"

Dr. James: (getting concerned): "You know, the Arter-Rooter XL? The big green one you take for your bad cholesterol, which is really, really, *super-duper* high?"

Mr. Smith (still affably, with a dismissive wave of his hand): "Oh THAT. Never took it."

Now Dr. James has several choices. He can:

1. Lunge across the room and wrestle Mr. Smith to the floor until he more fully understands that his wife is in imminent danger of becoming a widow (doctor fantasy action sequence);

2. Gently explain (again) the risk/benefit ratio of taking the medication and address any concerns about potential side effects; or

3. Leave Mr. Smith alone and write "NON-COMPLIANCE" in big letters on his chart to keep himself from being sued should Mr. Smith have a massive heart attack.

Most doctors think the former and do the latter. Outside of the fact that patients expose themselves to unnecessary risk, the other major reason doctors hate noncompliance is that it's a perfect waste of their precious time and energy. At first it drives young doctors nuts. Later in their medical careers, they relax because they realize they can't save the noncompliant patient, and they allow him to hit rock bottom until he finally decides to wake up. It's an interesting place for a doctor to be, but it does preserve his sanity. Because when your doctor is insane, that's *super-duper* scary.

Another important way someone can become a bad patient is to openly admit they practice voodoo.

Many doctors trained in Western medicine, with its emphasis on data, facts, and scientific proof, tend to be uncomfortable in the realm of the supernatural. But voodoo *really* throws us off. I once had a voodoo-practicing patient who would not cut her toenails. She feared that if some nefarious person were in possession of her toenail clippings, they could do something really bad to her from afar. I tried to convince her that most truly nefarious people are after more lucrative spoils than toenail clippings, but she was unflappable.

Yet another way someone can be put in the bad patient category, albeit through no fault of his or her own, is to be a lawyer. I don't understand why there is such natural enmity between doctors and lawyers, beyond all that pesky getting-sued stuff. When I find out a patient is a lawyer, I exclaim, "Oh! You're a lawyer! How neat! What kind of law do you practice?" Interestingly, I've *never, ever* had anyone tell me they were malpractice lawyers. Do they fib? Are they taught to fib about that in law school? Where do the malpractice lawyers get their medical care from, anyway? Their doctors must make them sign special waivers.

SECRETS OF THE GOOD PATIENT CLUB

Now that you know what not to do, how do you become a stellar patient? One of those patients who, when your doctor sees your name on her schedule, causes her to leap for joy? Well, the first thing is to act normally. If your doctor sees you being too ingratiatingly pleasant or complimentary, she'll suspect you're up to something.

The next thing is to let her talk as much as she wants. Doctors like to hear themselves talk, even though technically this is your visit. Doctors spend so much time fixing everybody else's problems that rarely do they get to air their own. I realize that doing this is risky, and possibly is like you going on a really bad blind date. Remember those? When the other person talked about himself or herself the whole time and you thought you'd have a seizure? And you wished you *would* have one, just so the date could end? (Your bad date *might* not have chased the ambulance.) But just listen. Your doctor will love you.

One last tip: Even when your doctor is running an hour behind, be patient and sweet with her, even though you may have reached your boiling point internally. She will remember you as "the really nice" patient, because the rest of the folks on her schedule gave her a hard time, one after the other after the other. If you do this, I thank you from the bottom of my heart. You are *such* a nice patient.

Helpful Guidelines for Sick Folks

I include this here because many people don't know what to do with themselves when they start to feel under the weather. I won't bore you with the obvious, like "go and lie down somewhere," "keep your hands washed," and "try not to cough all over pregnant women, elderly people, and babies." But here are a few pointers which may prove profitable:

1. *Admit that you need help.* This sounds simple, but for many folks it's not. It amazes me when people are sick but flatly deny that they have a problem and need help. Coughing up a lung and stumbling about in denial is completely counterproductive.

2. *Avoid toxic people who will derail your healing.* I was caring for a poor woman who had multiple huge abscesses in her legs. On one of her follow-up visits, her husband accompanied her. He watched silently as I unpacked and repacked her deep wounds; he saw her discomfort throughout the procedure. I'm sure he witnessed firsthand how miserable these things were for her every single day. So, logically at the end of the visit, he finally spoke up and said, "Doc, I just wanna know how soon she can have, you know, relations?"

Some people are difficult enough for you to deal with when you're healthy.

3. *Laugh as much as possible.* Immerse yourself in lighthearted books (like this one!), nothing too intellectual or too heavy to hold. Watching funny things on TV and reading cartoons are good ideas too. Laugh out loud until your family starts considering taking you back to the doctor for a recheck!

4. *Go ahead, eat some chocolate.* Of course having permission to eat chocolate is poorly timed, because when you're really sick you don't feel like eating anything at all. But try your best.

5. *Creatively engage friends and loved ones.* This is an excellent opportunity to have people do nice things for you. Has your car needed waxing for years? How about that brass bed that needs polishing? Certainly you would feel so much better convalescing in a beautiful, shiny bed instead of a crummy one, right?

6. *Take time to assess your life.* Mentally review the unfortunate stuff you wish you had done differently in life. Are you where you need to be with God? Do you need to make changes or patch things up with family members?

Illness can prompt us humans to refocus on what is truly important.

7. *Make a list of all the exciting things you're going to do once you're well.* Dreaming is healthy and good for the soul. In your mind's eye, picture yourself doing things you've never had the guts to do before. Go ahead—picture yourself driving a Harley, skydiving, or wrestling an alligator. Just make sure you picture yourself being successful!

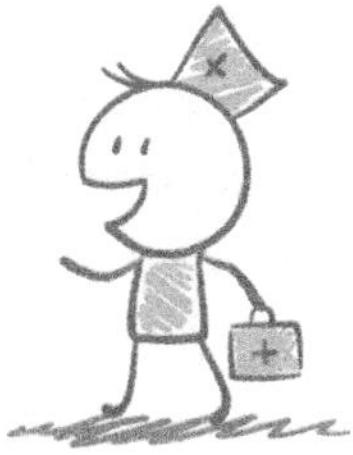

CHAPTER 7

WHEN YOUR PANTS ARE TOO TIGHT

IT'S THAT TIME AGAIN—when you, against your better judgment, go to reach for that pair of jeans in the closet. You're in a hurry and don't have time to be picky. The last time you tried this stunt, they were way too small. Hopelessly too small. "But maybe this time will be different," you think. Maybe the last time was a fluke. Maybe you've lost a little weight since then. Maybe Martians landed in your closet and . . . well, the possibilities are endless.

A tiny little voice pleads in your ear: "Don't do it! Don't do it!" But it's too late. Your big toe has already gone past the point of no return. Then it's all thighs, butt, and gut from then on, spilling, rolling, flopping out. The sheer horror of it all—those pesky Martians can't be trusted.

When I was growing up, having a little extra "meat on your bones" was a sign that you were blessed to have enough to eat. "Think about all those starving children all around the world," I was told as my plate was piled high. Thank the Lord for plenty. But in our current culture of carbohydrate-loaded, super-sized, fried overabundance and sedentary, overstressed overwork, we have a *big* problem. Literally. And no, we doctors are not immune. Many physicians are overweight. So the bulk of us are in the same boat. (The cool thing about doctors is that we're experts in giving really good advice that most of us don't follow and coming across as completely sincere. Neat, huh?) Some of our healthier medical colleagues run marathons and drink thirty-eight glasses of water a day, but the rest of us bums shun them.

Keeping Your Rear End Off the Evening News

When it comes to weight, here is the most important piece of advice I can think of: absolutely, positively, under no circumstances let your guard down and allow the local news station to video your rear end for their latest news report on obesity. That has to be one of the worst situations ever! And don't they prey on the most unprepared people? The ones who just happen to be caught out of the house in bright purple spandex pants? And yes, I realize that some of you insensitive readers do not feel that the words "just happen" and "spandex" go together. But it's been known to happen to many well-intentioned people.

I hope they give those poor people lots and lots of money. How would you feel if you were sitting down in front of the TV with a hamburger and fries and then, as you were savoring the first delicious, greasy bite, you saw your backside stretching all the way across your TV screen? Inevitably, those kinds of shots linger, because they have to get a prolonged shot of you walking down the street so that all the lumps of fat on your butt are jumping around at the same time.

That's one of the few things I remember from getting a chemistry degree: that oscillating Jell-O-like activity is termed "Brownian Motion." But even this special knowledge wouldn't comfort you in that moment of crisis. What would you do? Go into hiding? (I would, because I'd be certain that the whole world would recognize that particular rear end as mine.) Refuse to leave the house forever? Initiate legal action? That's more like it. I mean, if you can sue someone for libel, just think of the consequences for rear-end defamation! The more critical issue is whether or not you'd finish your burger. So watch your backside. Don't become a victim.

Finally, Some Good News about Extra Weight

Have you noticed that the medical profession blames every health problem on being overweight—heart attacks, cancer, diabetes, hypertension, lung disease, fatty liver, global warming? It's similar to when a smoker comes into the office saying, "I'm tired of you doctors saying all my problems are caused by smoking!" Well, they are, *so there.* Unfortunately, excess weight can have the same kind of impact on the entire body. Add back pain, hip pain, knee pain, and infections to the list above, and you end up with a whole batch of difficulties far too depressing to talk about in this book.

Since this is a happy book, let's try to find some *good* things about being overweight for a change. Babies and children like it—they have nice, soft places to pass out on. A few folks will admit they're physically attracted to fat, but they're statistically few and far between, or undercover, so you can't depend on them. If you happen to fall down, you're less likely to do damage to your internal organs, but if you fall on another person they may not fare as well. And the ultimate benefit: if there is a food shortage, you'd be a survivor, right? The runway models would be the first to go, right? But if things got really bad people might try to eat you first, so perhaps this is not a benefit after all.

How to Lose Weight

I've read about people who have come to accept being overweight as part of their identity. They claim they love being fat. Come again? I've no idea what those folks are talking about. Personally, I've been battling overeating and being chubby, overweight, and fat all my life. And I will likely continue to do so until I get to heaven, where I pray there will be lots and lots of chocolate. If you are overweight and have come to embrace fat, more power to you. I'm not there. I want my fat gone!

If you're like me, and you feel uncomfortable lugging more of you around than is necessary, what do you do? Deep down inside, you know that a major life change is probably needed.

But far too often, major change is only spurred by the need to lose weight quickly. Do you have a vacation coming up and need to fit into those swim trunks? How about an upcoming wedding? A twenty-year high school reunion? People who haven't seen you in decades will be analyzing every ripple, every jiggle. At least that's what I hear. I didn't dare go to mine.

People constantly ask me the best way (they usually mean the *fastest* and *easiest* way) to lose weight. If I were writing this just a few years ago, my fast, easy, and solitary answer would've been: diet and exercise. If more calories are consumed than are needed, the body is programmed to store the extra as fat. I still truly believe that healthy and sustained weight control absolutely depends on a lifelong commitment to three things: (1) eating a lower-carbohydrate diet rich in vegetables, with some lean protein and fruit, (2) exercising most days of the week, and (3) eating only when hungry and stopping when full. Getting plenty of sleep and play help a great deal as well. This does work, at least in part. I've seen this intuitive way of eating help me, my family members, and countless patients time and time again. Diet and exercise can be extremely difficult, but it's pretty straightforward. And outside of an occasional header off the treadmill, it's risk-free.

But over the last few years, obesity science has exploded. We are starting to understand more about how fat works. So, now my answer to how to lose weight is, "Diet and exercise…AND, it depends." Like everything else in medicine, it depends on many different factors, and not everyone is the same. Just as doctors don't just use one blood pressure pill to treat the thousands of patients they see with hypertension (although that would actually make their days go a lot faster), successful long-term weight loss requires that same individualized approach as well.

For some of us, including myself, excessive caloric intake comes from disordered eating.

Disordered eating is often born out of family dynamics and expands in the realm of the spirit, the hidden man. Excessive stress, guilt, self-hatred, boredom, anger, and fear (of failure, intimacy, being alone, attractiveness, other's opinions, lack, etc.) are often deeply hidden culprits. These need to be flushed out and healed. Even if medical technology were able to produce a totally risk-free medication or procedure for guaranteed permanent weight loss, those unaddressed areas of emotional need would simply manifest themselves in other ways, like shoe shopping. Which can be fabulous, by the way.

Surgery should not be a first option for those of us who eat emotionally. Certainly there are people who are severely obese and dangerously close to death who need to lose weight immediately. Any medical advance that may help save lives is greatly welcomed. But we who struggle emotionally with our food first need concrete mental, emotional, physical, and spiritual help and support. Anyone who has "heard" chocolate cake calling her after a break-up knows what I'm talking about. Anyone who, after a long and bitter day at work, comes home and rips open a whole bag of chips and shoves them frantically down his gullet knows what I'm talking about. We emotional eaters need to learn how to eat more normally by seeking peace for ourselves.

In addition, we know now that regular consumption of certain foods triggers this so-called hedonic eating. Regularly scarfing down high-fat, high-sugar, and high-salt foods can lead to wanting more and more of them. Dopamine, a major pleasure hormone, is released, which soon leaves us seeking our next "hit."

This is a great time to mention one of the most wonderful things known to man. Or woman. This, of course, is chocolate. Chocolate is a stimulant. In fact, medical literature suggests that it may stimulate the same areas in the brain as street drugs. But I disagree with the stigma of this comparison—chocolate is critical for maintaining lawful society by keeping its members sweet and sane. So for the sake of humanity, I refuse to stop eating it unless I become intensely and seriously allergic to it in an anaphylactic-shock type of way. I plan to eat chocolate until I draw my last breath. Ever choke on a piece of chocolate? And as you're choking and gasping for air, think to yourself, "Well, *this* is a fitting end"? I have. Food addiction is real. I can safely say that a diet high in carrots will not increase the risk of future carrot binges. But who really *wants* to binge on carrots?

Whether or not emotional eating is at play and to what degree, is a critical factor for physicians to consider when devising a weight-loss treatment plan.

Diets Don't Work

Okay, diets *do* work. But something very mysterious happens after you start losing weight. Here you are walking, squatting, doing sit-ups and jumping jacks, burning it up in Zumba class, and avoiding food like the plague for days and weeks and months on end. And you're looking good, getting compliments, and fitting into your old clothes really nicely. You're doing so well, you think, "This little tiny piece of cake won't hurt me—I've exercised today," or, my personal favorite, "I deserve this—I've worked so hard."

You start eating more "normally" just a few times a week for a few months, and something devilish happens to you: you wake up one morning and your "skinny clothes" don't fit. The weight that you so painstakingly lost has crept insidiously back on you like a ninja. You sigh deeply and haul out the "fat clothes" again. Believe me, I know. I've been up and down the scale ever since I was 5 years old, and I'll likely be battling weight until they lay my chubby body down.

Why do some of us battle so? How much can we possibly blame on genetics and physiology?

Are Your Genes Affecting Your Jeans?

If you're solidly-built like me, you've already accepted that you're not going to be a runway model. But are some of us destined to be fat?

Well, did you know that you are genetically programmed to have a certain number of fat cells from childhood through adulthood? And certainly most of us gain more fat cells over time. That means the gang of them that may be around your middle right this very second will never leave you nor forsake you! Of course, old fat cells naturally "turn over" and die, but they are replaced by new, fresh, eager ones. Now, before you throw yourself headlong into a bag of Oreos in despair, it gets worse. All you can do with your fat cells is shrink them, so just as easily as they've shrunk, they can just as easily pump up full of fat again. BAD fat cells! This is why "Lipo," total fat cell obliteration via laser, ultrasound, or good old-fashioned surgical suction, has become so popular. Extremely popular.

As far as a genetic basis for obesity, a sizeable number of genes have definitely been found to increase susceptibility to obesity, as well as where fat is deposited on the body. We also know members of various racial groups can have genetic predispositions to obesity. However, current thinking is that a mutation or deletion in a single gene is not the sole cause of an individual's weight, and the genes found so far may only explain a low percentage of obesity in the world's population as a whole. Diet and exercise (or lack thereof) have been shown to have the power to alter genetic risk, for good or for evil. Stay tuned; more to come. Until that time, at least we now do have a dim green light to continue to blame random family members for our lumpiness.

We're Just Learning about Fat

Whenever medical researchers think they're onto something good, they come to realize that they've only discovered the tip of the iceberg. The human body is so much more complex than they imagined, and they typically have to go back to the drawing board. Go figure. So when they discover a chemical target in the body's processes and then direct a drug toward that one part of the process, something else further down the chain can get messed up. That's why some drugs turn out to be lemons. They end up trading one bad thing for another because the whole process is not understood in its totality. But the good news is that researchers are learning more and more about how fat works as time goes by.

Now that we're in science mode, you might as well learn some technical jargon. That spare tire around your waist (you know, the "muffin top") is officially called *adipose tissue,* and fat cells are officially called *adipocytes.* But don't you like *fat cells* better? I do—it sounds more visceral, more raw. It makes reality come into focus extremely quickly.

Scientists are learning that fat is metabolically active. That means your fat cells don't just sit there, taking up excess space and wrecking your life. They actually produce inflammatory chemicals, called *adipocytokines,* that are also wrecking your life. And the more fat you have, the more inflammatory chemicals are produced. Bad news.

And not only do fat cells create inflammation, they produce chemicals that tell your brain what to do. Literally. You think your brain is the boss, it being the brain and what-not. But it looks like fat rises to the top once again. "I'm the boss of you," it sneers.

Fat cells produce a chemical called leptin, whose job it is to knock on our brain and inform it that we're full. When genetically obese, leptin-deficient lab mice were given leptin, they didn't eat as much and lost weight. But people who are medically obese have high leptin levels. Why? We can only speculate they may have some special resistance at the leptin protein binding site, or that their leptin binding sites don't work properly. In any case, it becomes harder for these patients to control their appetite and weight, simply because the brain remains clueless that the body's indeed satisfied.

Additionally, when folks lose weight, their leptin levels decrease, which increases hunger. This is one really important reason folks can gain back the weight they previously lost. Who knew? Most of us just thought we were horrifically weak-willed. So doctors can no longer presume how much hunger their overweight patients experience, nor condescendingly write them off as pitifully lacking self-control.

Just as leptin controls satiety, or the feeling of fullness, ghrelin is a hormone produced in the stomach that helps regulate hunger. It is elevated when we haven't eaten, but also interestingly when we don't get enough sleep. Think of ghrelin like a little gremlin that pokes and needles you into raiding the refrigerator at 11 o'clock at night. That's why doctors need to address sleep issues in their patients who struggle with their weight. If we can help our patients get better sleep, weight loss is facilitated.

There are many other hormones involved in hunger, satiety, and weight, and lots more to be discovered. Doctors now have a number of prescription medications at their disposal to potentially help selected patients who are very overweight and/or have health effects from their weight, provided they are appropriate candidates.

Because obesity is such a complex disorder, folks can find themselves literally trapped in a complex web of environmental, emotional, genetic, and hormonal factors that complicate their weight loss journeys. Obesity is now seen as a disease, and justifiably so. But as with all things, there is hope. We all do what we can, where we can, and how we can. Medical science will eventually catch up.

Your Body Mass Index (BMI)

Weight problems aren't necessarily always about having too much fat. If you don't have *enough* fat, you aren't healthy either. (Didn't your grandma berate you about being underfed and skinny when you were growing up? It's probably partially her fault you're in the mess you're in today.) An interesting medical study was published some years ago linking your body mass index (BMI) to your risk of dying. It was, as you can imagine, incredibly depressing.

But before we talk about the results of the study, let's calculate your BMI just for fun. "I'd rather have a root canal," you say. Don't be a chicken.

Take your weight in pounds, divide it by your height in inches twice, and multiply times 703. (Weight in pounds / height in inches/ height in inches x 703.) That number serves as a rough estimate of whether or not your weight is appropriate to your body size. (The number is not as useful if your muscles are well-chiseled chunks rippling across your body, but for the rest of us chumps it does okay.) Let's see where you are.

BMI Below 18—"The Stick Zone"

Eat something *now*. Start with a big, greasy hamburger and follow it immediately with a big, fatty milkshake. Doctor's orders. And no purging. Here's why: that medical study I just mentioned also showed that an underweight person's risk of dying from any cause is higher than that of a person with normal weight. Interesting, huh?

HOW TO GAIN WEIGHT

It always tickles me when thin people come to the office wanting a pill to gain weight. Most of these well-intentioned folks have no concerning medical illness; they just want more meat in the right places. Trust me on this one. You don't need a pill—you can do this the natural way. The key to gaining weight is to eat when you're not hungry. The operating plan is simple: develop an intense fear of hunger pains. Even if you've just eaten, desperately shove some cookies in your mouth on the off-chance that you *might* get hungry later. At least it's worked for me.

BMI 18–22—"The Normal Zone"

This range is thought to represent a healthy weight. The rest of us are secretly jealous of you. The only problem with being in this zone is that the risk of going out of bounds as you, ahem, get older is high.

To make our golden years even more enjoyable, researchers have gleefully pointed out that our daily caloric requirement decreases as we age because our metabolic rate falls like a brick. That means that even though we might've been watching our weight all our lives, when we're elderly and deserve to relax in the diet department, we actually have to up the ante. I don't know about you, but I was hoping to eat all the cinnamon rolls I wanted as I hurtled toward my final breaths—especially if I were already battling arthritis, ungrateful children, and a fixed income. Oh well.

BMI 23–29—"The Baby Fat Zone"

This is where those of you who have been trying to lose your "baby fat" since birth hang out. And women who have given birth and have still not dropped back down to their prepregnancy weight—even though their youngest child is now in college—may be here too. The medical community says you're officially overweight when your BMI is 25 to 29. Thanks! And as if that isn't bad enough, remember that incredibly uplifting study I was telling you about? It said that even though you may be only ten to twenty pounds overweight, your risk of dying from any cause is actually increased over your normal-weight counterparts.

When I read the study, it blew me away. Heart attacks, strokes, sure; embarrassment from having to wear a bathing suit, sure. Those I could understand. But your risk of checking out from, let's say, getting hit by a car while crossing the street is higher just because your BMI is higher? You'd think you'd be easier to see, being larger and all. Honestly.

BMI 30 and Up—"The Definitely Time-to-Take-Action Zone"

Our lovely friends the scientists have officially slapped you with the "obese" label when you find yourself here. But beyond the sheer pain of name-calling, this is where all those horrible health effects you're constantly barraged with on the nightly news come into play. It's time to make a concerted effort to lose weight. The good news is that small amounts of lost weight bring you further and further from the precipice of poor health. And you don't need to lose a hundred pounds to be healthier than before. Losing 5–10 percent of your body weight is an excellent start to help your body look, feel, and function better.

So how did you do? What are your next steps? Whether you're underweight, overweight, or in a good weight range, how can you maximize your health? I encourage you to talk to your doctor and set some reasonable goals with timelines to do so. You can do it! And I remain on the journey with you too.

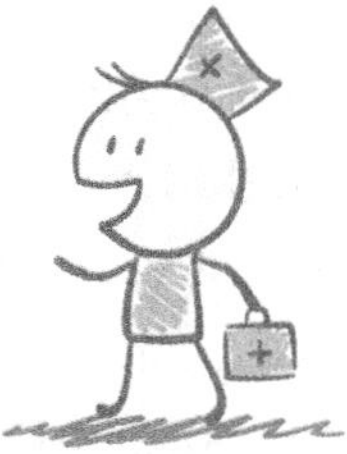

CHAPTER 8

WHAT YOUR DOCTOR THINKS ABOUT YOUR MEDICAL AILMENTS

The longer I practice medicine, the more convinced I am there are only two types of cases: those that involve taking the trousers off, and those that don't.

—Alan Bennett

YOU THOUGHT I MEANT to write "What Your Doctor Will *Do*" about them. Nope! We're going deeper. It's important to understand how your doctor thinks, because that will guide what he does.

I was in the supermarket once when a patient I knew ran excitedly over to me. In the middle of the bread aisle, he pulled up his shirt, pointed to his belly button, and asked, "Doc, I got this pain right here—what is it?" As if I were all-knowing! Truthfully, in the bread aisle I had no idea what might have been wrong with him, nor was I likely to guess without a complete understanding of his symptoms and associated symptoms, plus a physical exam and likely some tests.

I was tempted to be a smart aleck and respond, "Well, it sounds like you either have gas or your aorta is about to explode. Have a nice day!"

But I didn't. There are patients who hang on to a doctor's every word and accept each one as gospel truth. The real truth is that we doctors are human. In our minds, it's odd when people don't understand that we don't and can't know everything.

It's likewise amazing that some people not only invest doctors' words with profound meaning, but our barely audible grunts as well. Let's say your doctor asks you to open up your mouth and say "Ah." She shines her light in there and starts looking around. Then she starts frowning and making this concerned sound over and over, "Humm . . . huuumm." You start getting worried. Maybe she's discovered some horrible, cancerous growth in your mouth you knew nothing about (or you've got bad breath—one of the two).

What you don't know is this: She just remembered that she has to trudge to a parent-teacher conference tonight because her seven-year-old son, Billy, put a big wad of gum in a girl's hair and called her a "freckle face," and if he spent less time over at her ex-husband's house, little Billy probably wouldn't have these issues. Be reassured. Your doctor has already assessed that your mouth is normal. She's just drifted off for a brief second. Surgeons probably never have this happen, right?

On the flip side, other patients are starting to question everything we say—they prefer believing the evening news, random family members, and questionable sites on the Internet. But I'm not bitter. The public is becoming better educated about medical issues, which makes for fairly interesting office visits:

Patient (proudly shuffling an impressive stack of papers): "Thanks so much for seeing me today. As you can see, I've been on the Internet . . ."

Doctor (thinking to himself): "Uh-oh."

Patient: ". . . and I wanted to ask your opinion about this new robotic option I saw for hair growth. It was on *60 Minutes* last night."

Doctor (clueless and silently angry with his multiple medical journals for omitting the *real* issues he needs to stay current on): "Um . . . tell me what you know so far."

Patient: "Well, I'm just learning about it, but from what I understand, nanobots are injected into the hair follicles on your head and biochemically stimulate the follicles by enhancing the expression of the alpha-beta-5-turfbuilder isomerase gene. Could you please explain more about what happens after that step?"

Doctor (reduced to a pile of drool): "Duuuuh . . ."

We doctors like our patients to be educated. It's good, and it's healthy. But most of us also long for the days where we could just prescribe some penicillin and make everybody happy.

Medical technology and drug development are moving at breakneck speed. Especially if you're a doctor who cares for the whole body, keeping up with the latest and greatest for all the body's organs and all the different diseases is an incredible challenge. It's especially difficult when many brand-new developments are highlighted and advertised on TV or in home catalogs. New drugs, devices, and diagnostic tests may be years and years away from practical and ordinary use, but they do make good news. And most of us doctors don't have time to watch TV. We're feverishly trying to stay current with our medical journals, and what makes the medical news on TV is often very different from what's reported in our journals. For example, a patient once asked me if he should purchase a new home device for hemorrhoids that utilized electric currents. As you might imagine, home hemorrhoid electrocution had not yet made it into the formal medical literature. And though I had never heard of it, I could safely advise him that it sounded like a really bad idea.

What do you do if your doctor has no idea about the drug or procedure or herbal miracle you'd like more information about? If your doctor offers to research it for you, let him. If he offers to refer you to someone else for further discussion, let him. Just try not to give him a huge stack of information printed off the Internet to read. He's awfully busy and will be stunned into complete inaction. It might sit on his desk for months. Okay, years.

Doctors' Thoughts on Selected Ailments

The Big One

What's the most common thing people go to their doctor's office for? C'mon, guess! "Flesh-eating bacteria?" you say. Nope! "A rash?" you say. Try again! "Side effects from their medications?" Not bad, but nope! No indeed, one of the most common reasons patients come to see the doctor is (drum-roll, please): *a cold.* I kid you not. I am continually struck by this, even after sixteen years of practice. Many of my colleagues have just accepted this as a fact of life and moved on, but I continue to wonder why.

When *I* was growing up, kids didn't go to the doctor at all, except (maybe) to get their shots—it cost money. I still have this big scar over my right wrist from running through a glass door when I was five. I remember lots and lots of bleeding. "Just put some pressure on it!" still rings in my ears today. A few stitches would've been nice.

Back then when you got a cold, you got in bed, coughed and hacked and moaned a lot (the moaning was for special emphasis), and—the one bright spot—got to drink your grandmother's special alcohol-based "tea." Grandma's "tea" was a happy part of being sick. (Some of you, when your grandmother made her special cold remedy, never got to feel toasty and happy. You only got a smelly brew of onions, cod liver oil, and raw eggs with some green stuff floating around in it. Sorry.)

Fast-forward to the twenty-first century, and people are coming to doctors because they have colds. Eighty percent of those folks are absolutely convinced they have a sinus infection and want an antibiotic. Some of them are correct; a greater number are not. The remaining patients just want a pill to make all of their symptoms go away immediately. One patient, just six hours into a head cold, said that if she didn't feel completely back to normal in twenty-four hours, she'd be giving me a call. I explained to her that symptoms from an average cold last about a week or more, and that if I could cure the common cold, I'd be a gazillionaire. As expected, she gave me a call the very next day.

This truly is a microwave generation. Folks want everything done yesterday, and can't tolerate . . . well, anything. Their lives move too quickly to be slowed down by some dumb old virus. When a patient truly has a cold, what can doctors do? We can empathize, suggest some medications to reduce symptoms, and give advice: "Drink lots of liquids, and don't forget to drink some of Grandma's tea!"

Dizziness

You feel dizzy, unsteady, and lightheaded. You go to your doctor to get some straight answers. Or so you think. The trouble is that doctors, by and large, can't stand dizziness. There are three main reasons why, and it's not because they don't care about you or don't want you to feel better.

First of all, dizziness, like headache, is one of those symptoms that can come from a completely benign cause. But alternatively, it could be something *bad,* so doctors have to pay attention and listen carefully to you. That requires time, which is in incredibly short supply. The impetus to refer you to a specialist is incredibly strong for those docs who have three patients scheduled in a single fifteen-minute time slot.

The second reason docs may dislike this symptom is that patients have a hard time describing exactly what they're feeling, which is critical for an accurate diagnosis. Want to really aggravate your doctor and have her throw cotton balls at you? Be vague.

Now, in all fairness, the frustration can go both ways:

> *Doctor:* "Well, Mrs. Smith—Nurse Tina says that you've been feeling lightheaded lately?"
>
> *Mrs. Smith:* "No, Doctor. I haven't been lightheaded, I've been dizzy."

Doctor: "What exactly do you mean?"

Mrs. Smith: "You know, like I'm really, really dizzy."

Doctor: "Do you feel as if you're spinning or the room is spinning?"

Mrs. Smith: "I don't know—I'm just dizzy!"

Doctor: "Have you felt like you're going to pass out?"

Mrs. Smith: "Yes, yes, whatever. Just fix it!"

Doctors are looking for red flags, symptoms which tell us that you shouldn't leave the office under your own power. It takes patience—again, *time*—to get the job done properly.

Lastly, dizziness is such a sticky wicket for your doctor because even after doing an extremely thorough history, physical examination, and selected tests, he still won't be able to tell you the reason for your dizziness half of the time. Doctors like diagnostic slam dunks. Many of us are stalwart perfectionists who dislike not fixing problems, admitting uncertainty, or (a major issue) looking like fools. Starting out with a 50-percent failure rate is sobering. What keeps us going is the hope that in a slew of "dizzy" patients, we will find that one patient with a brain tumor, serious arterial blockage, or a heart valve problem. That's what it's all about. And making you feel better, of course.

Chest Pain

In contrast to dizziness, doctors like chest pain, because it's usually more clear-cut. In a doctor's mind, easier is better. And if you dare complain of chest pain, you will have some sort of heart evaluation no matter what, even if you're in the office for a hangnail. If you innocently mention to a fellow patient in the waiting room that you had chest pain two years ago after foolishly eating a huge greaseball "perfect storm" type of meal, you may find yourself whisked into the back of the office pronto. Doctor's offices have hidden microphones for those kinds of things. Even if it was a clear-cut spell of gas, you *will* have an EKG, and quite probably a stress test. If they're normal, we'll relax a bit.

Bad Teeth

Medical doctors don't understand why patients come to them for tooth pain. I didn't pay much attention to the one-hour dentistry lecture I had in med school, because I was attempting to focus on the rest of the human body. I assumed the dentists had teeth fairly well covered.

But I *do* know that green and black are typically bad colors for teeth to be. So when some poor suffering soul ends up in the office in torment from their green and/or black teeth, I just sit there, incredulous. I think to myself, "What do they want me to do? I'm not a dentist." Then I explain that the only method of real, lasting toothache relief I know to provide involves tying one end of a string to their bad tooth and the other end to a doorknob and slamming the door as hard as possible. Surprisingly, no one's taken me up on my offer of treatment yet, even though it's far cheaper than your typical extraction.

Pain

Pain is the signal that your body sends you when something is wrong with it, like when you accidentally sit on a tack. Your body says, "Hello! Sharp pointy thing here! It's really sharp!" Wouldn't it be interesting if your body actually spoke audibly when you had pain? Some helpful comments your body might make:

Stomach: "Hey you up there! Would you mind slowing down on the hot wings?"

Elbow: "Excuse me, but would you please lay off the tennis and picking up your forty-pound kid for a little while? And the stomach wants me to tell you to slow down on the hot wings."

Overloaded knees (in concert): "Yo, Dude! You *definitely* need to slow down on the hot wings! Ditto the pizza, the cookies, *and* the Doritos!"

And on it would go. Either you would be amazingly fit, or driven insane by all the chatter.

As far as doctors' attitudes are concerned, some of us actually get irritated by pain complaints, even though it's a major reason people come to us. Unless patients have an obvious source of pain, like from cancer, surgery, or a bone broken in three places, it can be hard for doctors to wrap our minds around pain. We tend to comprehend poorly those things we can't see, feel, or measure.

Other hindrances doctors have regarding pain: (1) Some patients' organs work just fine, but their pain is a result of emotional trauma; (2) Some patients' pain is due to a difficult-to-diagnose problem that has yet to be figured out; and (3) Some patients pretend to be in pain so they can obtain narcotic pain medication. These last folks make doctors defensive and guarded in their approach to treating pain. Once doctors have had multiple bad experiences with drug-seeking patients, they become very wary. Unfortunately, this makes it difficult for some people with legitimate pain to be viewed objectively.

Bleeding

Doctors like blood, even internists—up to a certain point, of course. It means something is measurably wrong. If you tell a doctor you're bleeding, your predicament becomes strangely more interesting for her than if you're "only" having pain, especially if your doctor is a surgeon.

> *Patient:* "Doctor, I'm having this pain in my belly."
>
> *Surgeon* (anticipatingly): "Are you noticing any . . . *bleeding* perhaps?"
>
> *Patient:* "Why yes! How did you know?"
>
> *Surgeon* (excitedly to himself: "JACKPOT!"; and gravely to the patient): "We've got to take care of this right away!"

Bleeding puts you into a different patient category altogether.

Another thing about bleeding: Some patients—not surprisingly, male ones—don't even bother mentioning it. I had this one man come in for a diabetic visit. As I was examining him, I noticed he had some blood on his sock. Incredibly astute clinician I am, I realized something was measurably wrong. I made him take his sock off despite his strong assertions that he was "fine." He had a huge, ugly ulcer on his foot that he had not apparently planned to bring to medical attention any time this century.

I could give scores more examples of doctors' mindsets relative to different medical complaints, but this would take all the mystery out of your next doctor appointment. Just know that your doctor certainly has deep thoughts beyond the regular medical nuts-and-bolts components of your case.

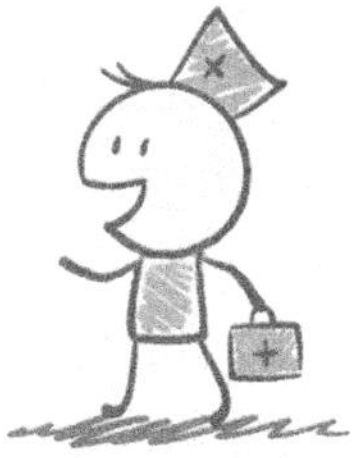

CHAPTER 9
PATIENT POTPOURRI

I went to the doctor and he said I had acute appendicitis. And I said, "Compared to who?"
—Jay London

IN THIS CHAPTER, we'll explore some of the specific medical challenges of guys, gals, and kids, and share some thoughts on getting older. The guys can go first so they don't find themselves accidentally in the midst of any menstrual-related content. I suspect that the gals will read this chapter in its entirety anyway.

GUY STUFF

The DRE

Let's start with the end in mind. The biggest source of stress and consternation for guys when they visit the doctor is having a prostate exam, what doctors call the DRE. Numerous urban legends prevail—that such an exam can cause the stoutest and bravest of men to be rendered unconscious, or that it can alter sexual orientation. Many guys completely avoid seeing the doctor over it, placing their health in great jeopardy.

DRE stands for digital rectal exam. And I probably just lost about half of the guys right there. You knew it was coming anyway, so let's let it see the light of day. There will be many derrière-related jokes to help lighten the mood. You've been fore-(and rear-) warned. See how many puns you can find.

The DRE is a way for doctors to directly assess the size and smoothness of the prostate gland in order to help diagnose an enlarged or cancerous prostate. And please note that men have a prostate gland, not a "prost*r*ate" gland. "Prostrate" is what you are *during* the DRE, which is defined per the Oxford Dictionary as "lying face downward, esp. in submission." Let's not get the terms mixed up.

Women do not have prostates. One lady patient once asked me to check hers, and she left the office disappointed. Older women do, however, get rectal exams too. Why? Because doctors also use DREs to screen for hidden blood, which may indicate colon cancer. So if you're a guy who is lucky enough to get a DRE, you're actually getting two cancer tests in one: a prostate test with a colon test bringing up the rear. How's that for a deal?

Despite its unfair reputation, the DRE is an important and medically necessary examination tool that all men must undergo by presidential order, starting at the very latest by the age of fifty (sooner if you have a family history of prostate cancer, are African-American, or per your doctor's preference)."Later for the president," you quip. But not so fast! I'm sure the President gets his rectal exam like everybody else, and that's one time he really wishes he didn't have the Secret Service hanging around.

Anyway, back to you. The whole reason we doctors attempt to give you a DRE seemingly at every opportunity is so we can make you feel as dehumanized as possible. Just kidding! Seriously, our intentions of trying to screen for prostate disease and colon cancer are noble ones. The end does justify the means!

How do you prepare yourself physically, mentally, and emotionally for your DRE? Personally, I'd like more guys to *bathe*. I had one man tell me, "If I knew you were gonna do all this, I would've taken a shower." Bathing before any doctor's appointment is always a good idea. Remember that your doctor's face will be down there, and even on a good day the view is anything but scenic.

Next, make sure you pick a doctor who has skinny fingers. This makes a huge difference. Whenever a man balks at me, a lady doctor, doing his rectal exam, I gently inquire if he would prefer my six-foot-three-inch, three-hundred-pound male colleague who was a defensive tackle during his college football days.

Thirdly, practice overcoming the biggest hurdle, which is fear of pain. Let me assure you—a rectal exam does not hurt. Do *not* listen to your buddy who tells you that he knew someone who knew someone who passed out while getting it. No guy has ever passed out when I did his rectal. If anyone did, the fainting spell was brief, I didn't notice it, and he left it behind him. It does not hurt! It just feels, well, strange. There is a vague sensation that something unusual is going on. It's doable. What's truly painful is having your body riddled with prostate cancer that's spread to your bones.

The last obstacle to conquer mentally is the concern that you won't look macho during the rectal. It's perfectly okay for guys to kick their ladies out of the exam room at that juncture. We understand: It's just not a cool position to be in. But it's also not macho to be up going to the bathroom six times a night because of an enlarged prostate either. So please don't let fear of embarrassment stop you from getting checked out.

Mojo Gone Missin'

Loss of libido is the second most common guy concern we doctors encounter. But this is a family book. So, I've made the executive decision not to delve into the universe of prescription pills and over-the-counter supplements available. Suffice it to say that if your female doctor tells you that blindness is one of the potential side effects of a medication, avoid loudly ranting that you'd rather go totally and utterly blind than not get a prescription. This is the one time she will likely have absolutely no ability to relate.

The second thing is this: Don't assume that "supplements" are automatically safer than prescription meds. Remember, supplements are not regulated and could contain *anything*. I could scrape the grass clippings off my lawnmower, grind them up, add food coloring, and market my concoction as "Super-Duper All-Natural Doctor-Recommended Manly-Man Love Extract" and make some *serious* money. (Hmmm . . .)

Recently, a number of supplements are being found to cause liver damage. So please discuss whatever you plan on taking with your doctor. Personally, I love it when guys come to me and ask me if an herbal product is "safe," especially when they've already been taking it religiously for the last six months.

And one final word about testosterone supplementation. It will be quick because I'm admittedly paranoid. I *know* that guys with low testosterone can feel great on it. I *know* that guys' lives can be changed. But it's as if the medical community didn't learn *anything* from giving women estrogen for decades on end. You see, years ago doctors liberally prescribed estrogen to every older woman who crossed their paths. We thought we were doing a good and noble thing. But over time we found out that doing so may increase a woman's risk of heart disease, breast cancer, and uterine cancer. Consequently, we've become judicious and selective about which women receive hormone replacement therapy and how long they're exposed to it.

These days, it's medically fashionable to replace testosterone in men. But we've been here before, and I fear we doctors are once again getting caught up in all the hype. We don't know the long-term effects of putting millions of older men on testosterone and exposing them to it for decades on end. We don't know how significantly testosterone supplementation may affect men's prostates long term. Consequently, I'm for judicious and selective replacement. Anytime we attempt to alter our bodies' physiology, new and unexpected challenges (side effects) arise. As with all drug treatments, the benefits should far outweigh the risks—because there *will* be risks.

COLONOSCOPIES FOR ALL

Colonoscopies are for both guys and gals over fifty years old and for younger folks who have any problems in that geographic region. A skinny, fiber-optic flexible camera is inserted up the rectum and way up, across, and down your large intestine. It's a powerful tool not only to diagnose colon cancer, but to spot other important bowel problems as well. It's true that medical science is evolving rapidly, and now they even have little cameras (pill endoscopy) that you actually swallow so your doctor can look at your innards noninvasively. But if those cameras find something, she's still got to lug the colonoscope out anyway to check it out further.

I personally believe you should be sedated for your colonoscopy. I've heard from many patients who have experienced the test with and without happy medicine, and I definitely give a nod to the value of being out of it. I assisted in a colonoscopy once where the nicely sedated, happy patient drowsily muttered, "Doc, can I have another one of these colon things?" You get the picture. And for an uncomplicated procedure, at the most you'll experience some gas afterward—you shouldn't experience any rectal pain.

There are some doctors out there who don't use conscious sedation for their colonoscopies. They just don't believe it's necessary. I suspect they're the same extremists who say docs don't need to use lubricating jelly when they do rectal exams. If you ever come across a doctor who won't give you anything for your colonoscopy, run! Better yet, you might want to back out of the room—just in case.

Girl Stuff

Ladies get most concerned about changes their bodies go through—especially the ones that make them look old. We already dealt with the whole gaining weight thing in an earlier chapter, so we'll skip that. We'll deal with getting old and wrinkled a bit later, so we'll skip that too. Let's talk about pregnancy and menopause, the two woman issues I have yet to personally experience. (Lack of personal experience *never* stops a doctor from putting her two cents in. How many oncologists have actually had chemo? How many male OBs have ever had a Pap smear? I rest my case.)

Pregnancy

If you're a pregnant woman, I am of absolutely no help to you. If you do happen to go into labor in my presence, I can dial 911 and boil water with the best of them. If pressed, I can even help catch the baby and tie and cut the umbilical cord (but when it's time to deliver the placenta, I'm out of there).

OB was the worst rotation for me in medical school—*worst* in the sense that I could never wrap my mind around that mystical, arcane science. Here's what would happen during my typical OB shift:

It's midnight on the "Labor Deck." All twenty birthing rooms are full, it's a full moon, and somehow nearly all the women, in exacting, bloodcurdling unison, are screaming in horrific pain. It's really creepy, and the ward sounds like a medieval torture chamber, despite new life coming into the world and all that. It promises to be a long night. I silently vow never to personally go through labor conscious.

Upper-Year OB Resident (in a cranky, sleep-deprived voice): "Go check Bed 12."

Me, the Newbie Medical Student (hearing "Bed 12" before I see her, a hard-faced, haggard woman clutching the bed rails in blatant distress): "Hello, Mrs. Brown? How are you feeling?"

Mrs. Brown (gaping at me incredulously): "What does it look like? AARRGGH!"

(I figure this is not the best time to compliment her on her excellent pirate impression.)

Me (running to get the resident, who has wearily slumped in a chair): "Um, I'm not sure, but I think Mrs. Brown is in labor. Could you come take a look?"

Resident (sighing heavily and clearly annoyed at my ignorance): "How far along is she?"

Me (thinking, "There's *no way* I'm getting close enough to her to find out"): "Um, I would feel more comfortable if you checked her."

Resident (checking, irritated): "She's barely a centimeter. Tell her not to push."

Me: "Say what?"

Resident (growing more irritable): "I said, *tell her not to push.*"

Me (softly, apologetically, to Mrs. Brown): "He says not to push."

Mrs. Brown (loudly and irritably): "I've had two kids; I know when to push!"

Me (softly, apologetically, to resident): "She says she knows when to push."

And on it went. Such was the extent of my OB education—me being told what to say and do, even when it made no natural sense. The one part I loved was seeing the babies silently emerge, encased in slime and goo, and then morph into angry little warriors. I longed to go to the warmer and help welcome them into the world. Instead I was stuck delivering the placenta, stitching up tears in the birth canal, and dodging various bodily fluids that shot out in my general direction. Please don't get me wrong—the entire birthing process is a wonderful miracle and all, but I'd still rather go play with the baby. C'mon, you would too. Baby or placenta? You make the call.

So I was scarred for life after my OB rotation. I was dead set on not doing any more OB stuff *ever*, and I was safe during my internal medicine/pediatrics residency. When I got into practice, I handled pregnancy confirmation visits with aplomb ("Yup, you're pregnant!"). If a pregnant woman had a cold, ear infection, or something else really simple, I could see her without a problem. I even could (gasp) measure the baby's heartbeat with an ultrasound probe. Sometimes the mother would have to show me where to put the probe ("Um, Doctor, last time my OB did this she listened on the *opposite* side"), but I was quite proud of myself anyway.

Then, one fateful day, a pregnant patient somehow got on my schedule for a prenatal visit. At first I thought the staff was playing a joke. Then I realized that the woman was really pregnant, really sitting in my exam room, and had *real questions.* I didn't want to look like a complete and total wuss, so I went inside the room with her and (gasp) *closed the door.* All I could do was stare at her belly. I don't even remember her face. I was too busy nervously eyeballing her abdomen for signs of impending labor. You non-OB docs out there know exactly what I'm talking about!

Her first question to me was, "Am I gaining enough weight?" And me being the ignorant non-OB doctor that I am, I said "Sure!"(I mean, her belly was *huge.* I figured that if I couldn't wrap my arms completely around her, she was probably doing okay.) Then she told me she was having pain across her right flank, and asked, "Is this pain normal, Doctor?"

That was it. I was through. I lasted a whole 2.35 seconds. I had to go get one of my family practice colleagues who knew what they were doing. The staff and I had a mutually beneficial talk about that particular appointment later on that day.

Menopause

Menopause issues make up a sizable chunk of what ladies seek medical help for. It's not the lack of periods—most ladies are more than happy to do without that monthly drama. It's the weird symptoms that can go along with it that can be so very unsettling.

Take this quiz to see if you could be in menopause:

1. Are you a woman? Yes No

   (Actually, we now understand that middle-aged men have their own hormonal version of menopause called andropause—wives throughout history have *always* suspected something was going on.)

2. Are you over the age of 48? Yes No

   If not, you may need special blood tests to see if you're in "The Club." You didn't know there was such a thing? Well, it's like the Childbirth Club—once you go through labor, you're in. Menopausal ladies give each other knowing nods when they see each other breaking out in a full, glorious sweat.

3. Have you ever walked around in the dead of winter dressed in a tank top and shorts?

Yes No

If so, did you feel overdressed? Yes No

4. Are your husband and family suddenly agreeing to everything you say, even if it's something like, "Let's sell the house and join the circus?" Yes No

5. Have you ever had two fans blowing on you at the same time? Yes No

And do you think two fans are for lightweights?

Yes No

6. Are you getting an amazing amount of housework done at 3 a.m. because you can't sleep?

Yes No

Count each "Yes" answer as a point.

If you scored 4–6 points, congratulations! You're probably in The Club!

If you scored 1–3 points, you may be on your way, but you aren't fully there yet.

If you scored 0 points, what in the world made you take this quiz?

What Is Menopause, Anyway?

This special time is when your estrogen switch is in the process of going to the "off" position. *Menopause* sounds better than *menostop.* But it's misleading, because *pause* implies it will restart again, when in reality it's destined to stop, unless we doctors (da-da-dum!) decide to intervene.

For some ladies, this process is gradual and mild. Some lucky few even say they have no symptoms at all. They say they have a very pleasant experience, like a ride in the country on a sunny day. For other women, those hormones go down kicking and screaming, exorcist-style. If you're not there yet, how do you know which category you'll be in? One easy answer is to look at your mother. Personally, I'm in trouble. But you may be better able to manage if you're prepared.

Estrogen is an important hormone because it has so many effects on a whole bunch of really important organs. We know a lot about the bones, skin, heart, and certainly the girl equipment, but we're starting to look more closely at how the brain is affected too. Out of all the bothersome symptoms of menopause, ladies tend to ask the following questions:

"Doctor, is it normal to . . .

. . . feel like you're losing your mind?"

. . . not be able to get any sleep? At all?"

. . . occasionally wish your husband would go get lost in the woods?"

. . . forget really important stuff, like your wedding anniversary?"

With menopause, most anything is fair game in my book, because every woman is different. One medical study tried to define what symptoms could legitimately be attributed to menopause and which ones were suspect. For example, it refuted the age-old wisdom that menopause was associated with insomnia. Now, I'm just a little primary care doc, but I cannot count how many times women have come in to me for insomnia since they've hit menopause. They've never had problems sleeping before, ever. Which am I to believe? A medical study? Or all the women in my office begging for relief?

Another common issue is the difference between *hot flash* and *hot flush.* The medical literature favors the term hot flush. But I like hot flash because it underscores the aggressive intensity of the experience. Flush makes me think of something demurely feminine and fleeting, not something that can totally ruin a shower in two minutes and make your hair frizz up.

Once you and your doctor (and your husband and kids and friends and coworkers and random people on the street) are in agreement that you are, in fact, in menopause, the next big decision is treatment. Do you need drugs? Which kind? For how long? This is an incredibly sticky wicket, as you also have the bio-identical hormone devotees on one side and the synthetic estrogen advocates on the other. Please talk to your doctor. Don't be surprised when your doctor uses words like "We don't have much data on that," or "It's probably not a good idea for you," or "Maybe it's not the worst idea if you're homicidal; please don't hurt me." Good luck.

When Your Kid Is Sick

When your child is sick, it's always scary. Does your child just have a cold, or meningitis? I mean, *really.* And you're always hearing bad stories about so-and-so's kid who nearly died, even though he didn't even have a fever, because his trifling parents didn't take him to the doctor soon enough. Of course you don't want anything to be wrong with your child, nor do you want to be labeled a bad parent. So you take Little Johnny in to see the doctor.

As you're waiting in the exam room, something miraculous starts happening to Little Johnny. He starts getting inexplicably better. Here you were, at 2 a.m., wondering what in the world happened to your child, and by 9 a.m. he's ticklish and giggling, jumping and flailing about. What happened? I'll tell you: Magic air. Doctor's offices have this specially pumped in. You need to know this as a parent so that you won't feel so bad when the doctor raises her eyebrows at you when you tell her, "He was really sick before, honest!" So you get the clean bill of health, get to your car, buckle Little Johnny in, and he starts doing "it" again. I mean, *really.*

"It's Just a Virus"

Don't you just love this line? This is our doctor mantra. Doctors are taught to say this during their pediatric training; we have an "it's just a virus" quota to fill every day under the Hippocratic Oath. Here is a list of your child's symptoms that doctors will ascribe to a virus 98 percent of the time:

- Congestion
- Conjunctivitis
- Cough
- Diarrhea
- Fever
- Forgetting to tell you he brought a snake home and now he can't find it
- Headache
- Neglecting to tell you his science fair project is due tomorrow
- Rash

+ Runny nose
+ Sore throat
+ Vomiting

Does this sound familiar? And don't mention that your child is in day care—doctors will tell you it's a virus before you even finish saying the words.

So why is this? It's because viruses are ubiquitous—that means they're everywhere. In the air. On surfaces. On doorknobs and handles. On money. On toys. On your boss's hands when he gives you a handshake, because he was just picking his nose moments before (but you suspected that already). And when kids get these viruses they tend to pass them on to everyone in the house to ensure maximal family bonding. And there are *a gazillion* viruses out there. Neat, huh?

I have this "it's just a virus" spiel down pat: "Just because Little Johnny probably has a virus doesn't mean he's not sick, blah, blah, blah. It means that we don't have any medicines to kill the virus and make it go away, blah, blah, blah. If I could cure the common cold, I'd be rich, blah, blah, blah."

I know you as a parent have heard it all before. But better "just a virus" than something truly bad and ugly. Been there, done that. I've seen plenty of kids bad sick, and that is an awful place for them to be.

Getting Older

We all get there—that stage in our lives where our bodies start falling apart. It's normal, it's natural, it's inevitable, and it stinks. Previously faithful organs that you've relied on for decades begin to betray you and flatly refuse to obey the simplest command.

Let's say you're trying to fill out paperwork. The form asks you for your address, and for a split second you draw a total blank. The only thing you can come up with is where you lived ten years ago. You write your best guess down, but the words look strange on paper. Is that even the right zip code? What do you do when your own brain fails you miserably? Can you trust yourself to handle anything else?

If you want my advice, just chalk it up to a "busy brain" day. That's what I do. And it's perfectly legal to peek at your driver's license if you need a hint. Obviously, although I've had my moments, I'm not elderly yet. But as many older patients so graciously say, "You'll see!" Oh, joy.

I've already had some practice being elderly, thank you very much. On the first day of medical school we had to complete a patient simulation exercise. Students were randomly assigned certain tasks in a desperate attempt to teach us empathy for our future patients. For example, several male students had to don a flimsy paper gown and lie in gynecologic stirrups in an exam room for an hour with the air conditioning running full blast. (I'm guessing whoever thought of that exercise was not a guy.)

My own patient simulation exercise was to practice being elderly. Ill-fitting, thick glasses smeared with Vaseline were strapped to my head. My feet were bound to big heavy bricks of unequal height, and my back was laden with a large backpack full of, you guessed it, more bricks. Earplugs and a cane were shoved in my ears and my hand. My seemingly simple assignment was to walk a predetermined course around the campus in that stricken state.

As a fit and foolish twenty-one-year-old, I relished the challenge. That relish lasted ten whole minutes. Then I got weary. Weary of steps. Weary of long, flat stretches of concrete. Weary of no one holding doors open for me. Weary of not being able to see well, hoping I didn't fall over or get knocked down. Weary of saying, "Huh?" Weary of constant, nagging back pain. When the exercise ended, a tiny little nubbin of empathy had sprouted, but it was overwhelmingly overshadowed by relief that I could take all that garbage off. I merrily resumed being twenty-one and ragingly healthy again.

Now that I'm in my forties, this getting older thing is more personal. No longer can I just jump up and run a mile. I have to seriously warm up first—for about a month. Know what I mean? I own a heating pad, multiple bottles of analgesics, and several tubes of smelly muscle rub (and I don't even care that it's smelly). There are lots of new noises ("What was that, my hip?"), new aches and pains, new gray hair, new wrinkles, sags, and blotches, new dysfunctions, more doctor visits, more tests, and less overall cuteness. Right now, these changes are mildly amusing and occasionally expensive—but I'll see how it goes over time. I refuse to be scared. My plan is to develop a sparkling personality to compensate.

The potential for physical devastation aside, and assuming the mental faculties are still reasonably intact, there are a few things about getting older that are actually neat.

Wisdom

Granted, this is not guaranteed. Just because a person has gray hair does not mean he can make sound decisions or offer quality advice. But when we are older and wise, we can actually help young people. The big problem, as we already know, is that young people don't listen.

Freedom

People should be free to be themselves. Kids and older people are best at exercising this natural right. When a five-year-old boy decides to wear his favorite superhero underwear, he wears it and wears it confidently. Unfortunately, after childhood, we learn to care about what folks think or say. As we age, we usually unlearn this tragic tendency until we finally realize that people's opinions simply don't matter. When a seventy-five-year-old woman decides to take up waterskiing, she does it, regardless of how her family and neighbors might perceive her. Obviously we should be sensitive and considerate of others, but not at the expense of realizing goals and dreams that are planted inside of us by God.

Quality Choices

As long as our hearts are beating, we have the opportunity to decide every day whether to be happy or to be miserable. We have the choice to hang it up, roll over, and die, or to seize each day given to us with expectancy and hope. This is true no matter who we are or what our financial status might be. But it's especially critical as we age. We need to make more quality choices, because we have less time to get stuff accomplished. Our window of opportunity is smaller. As we see the finish line approaching, a holy fire can develop on the inside of us to burn off the chaff of the temporal and refine our hold on the eternal. What truly counts if we're near the end of our race? That we fulfill our individual purpose and calling during the short time that we're here.

I've seen many older people refuse to pursue purpose by stating, "I'm too old." Too old for what? Life? Age is no reason to opt out of being who you were created to be. And if you're physically too tired, at least do something, anything, toward your dream. You might find that acting on your dreams gives you extra energy you didn't even know you had.

If you are alive today, there's a reason why. God gave you breath today so you could be joyfully productive, not so you could wallow incessantly in regret, defeat, and self-pity. See the Epilogue for how to defeat that mindset. And if you've already made up your mind to maximize your life right up until you take your very last breath, congratulations! I'll see you at the finish line!

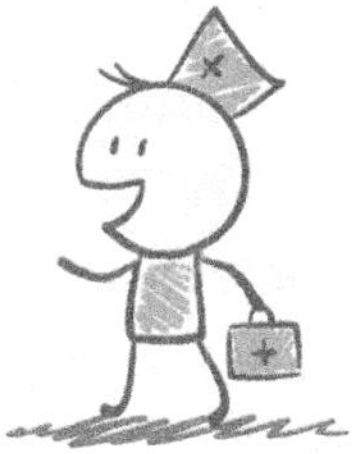

CHAPTER 10
THE SECRET LIVES OF DOCTORS

Like plumbing, medicine is a profession where you learn early on not to put your fingers in your mouth.
—Diana Gabaldon

NEWSFLASH—YOUR DOCTOR is just as goofy as you are. Goofy as in "leaves the TV remote in the refrigerator." Goofy as in "puts on mismatched socks." Goofy as in "loses her car in the parking lot." Because our family members could really get us in trouble here, we doctors have secretly sedated them for this chapter. We promise to wake them up later. Our nurses are too vigilant for us to sneak anything into their drinks, but we gave them the day off. So the information presented in this chapter will be glaringly biased and one-sided (not unlike the rest of the book).

What kind of person becomes a physician? We come in all types—some who are inexplicably insecure, others whose egos could fill a skyscraper. The bulk of us are regular people. As young children, some of us played with toy stethoscopes and found cures for all our stricken stuffed animals; others contentedly passed the time eating Play-Doh. We're not superhuman, nor are we infallible. We're just people who have decided to make a career out of hanging around sick people.

Doctor Wannabe Self-Assessment Test

Have you always wondered if you have what it takes to be a physician? I've met a number of people who deeply regret never taking the plunge. And I meet bright-eyed premed students all the time who typically have no idea what they're getting into. They have no doctors in their families, have never shadowed one, and naïvely think (exactly as I did) that doctoring would be a "pretty neat thing to do." All right then. Check off the appropriate boxes and tally your score.

Are you willing to:

- ❑ Go to school forever? At the very minimum, eleven years after high school?

- ❑ Earn really good grades while you're in school forever? This involves studying, which involves self-sacrifice on a recurring basis, such as not watching TV or going to parties or movies or the beach. Or having a life, really.

- ❑ Search your soul for one truthful and decent reason why you want to be a doctor? "I want to help people" won't get you through the first week of med school.

- ❑ Burden yourself, your family, and your spouse with massive amounts of debt that will take decades to pay off?

- ❑ Eat, sleep, talk, and be totally consumed by your job day in and day out during post-graduate training, which will last seven years or more?

- ❑ Get intensely personal with blood and guts and a whole plethora of other bodily emissions, all of which are fiercely unpleasant, especially if they get on you? Except baby drool—that's cute.

- ❑ Be physically, mentally, and emotionally unavailable to your spouse, children, family, friends, and even yourself for months and possibly years at a time?

- ❑ While on hospital call, forsake sleep, and frequently personal hygiene, for the greater good of the patient?
- ❑ While on call at home, answer critical life-and-death phone calls at 3 a.m. regarding foot fungus, nasal congestion, and hair loss?
- ❑ Take hugely stressful recertification exams all throughout your career until you drop dead, retire, or just stop being able to pass them, whichever comes first?
- ❑ Hone critical collateral skills in salesmanship, customer service, individual and couples counseling, homeopathy, personal training, drug rehab, mind reading, creative writing, begging, and eating crow?

How did you do?

If you checked off eight or more, you just might be twisted enough to make this medicine thing happen. Otherwise, I advise you to drop all med school fantasies, become truly productive by starting your own business doing something you enjoy, and make a positive intergenerational impact on your community.

LOOKING THE PART

We measure a doctor's competence by his dress, his brand of watch, and even the car he drives. This was my grandmother's attitude. "If he can't take care of his shoes, he can't take care of me!" was her undying motto. Although I agree that spit-shined shoes do make a fine impression, keep in mind that a doctor can be "tight" on the outside but not right on the inside. Hopefully there's more to a doctor, or any person for that matter, than meets the eye.

Let's assume you don't require your doctor to drive a BMW or Mercedes. But would you be concerned if he pulled up in a black-smoke-belching, rusted-out beast (where the word *car* itself would be a stretch), with taped-on plastic sheeting instead of windows? Would you be concerned because he doesn't care about his vehicle, and perhaps this apparent lackadaisical attitude might spill over into your medical care? Or, worse yet, that he's broke because he's lost one too many malpractice cases? Of course you would! Deep down inside, people do care what we look like, dress like, and drive.

Inquiring Minds Want to Know

Barring the basic "my doctor looks like/dresses like/smells like Frankenstein" concern, most patients truly don't care about the details of their doctors' personal lives. They simply want to make sure their doctors are halfway smart and fully sane. But for those of you who really want to know what we're like, here's a sample interview:

Q: *Dr. White, why did you become a doctor?*

A: I wanted to help people (Dr. Woodhouse paid me to say that). No, actually, I was tired of my family saying I'd never amount to anything, so this has pretty much kept them off my back.

Q: *What do you like most about being a doctor?*

A: I love all the extra attention I get, like my next-door neighbor asking me for a prescription for his arthritis.

Q: *You look like you're doing pretty well financially, Doc. What would you say is your financial motto?*

A: Here it is: "I'm in so much debt, I deserve a Benz." Did I mention that it's leased?

Q: *Do you really work out yourself, or do you just tell everybody else to?*

A: I ran cross-country before I went to med school twenty years ago, so I'm hoping that will tide me over until I retire.

Q: *How smart are you, anyway?*

A: I got a 1575 on my SATs, and I have an IQ of 140. But ask me why I'm still

$80,000 in debt and haven't really seen my wife for the last two weeks.

Q: *Are your kids just as messed up as everyone else's?*

A: I wish I could say that they weren't. My teenage daughter just went out and got this gigantic green tattoo on her neck after I told her not to.

Q: *How are you mentally, Doctor?*

A: I think I'm still in my right mind. You'd better ask my wife and kids, though—oh, I forgot, they're in the back, still heavily sedated for this chapter. I've got to make sure I check on them soon.

Q: *Would you do it again, if you had to live life over?*

A: You mean, get all those years back? Tough question. I went to med school when I was twenty-one years old. I don't know anything else, haven't learned any other trade. If I were replaced tomorrow, I wouldn't have the slightest clue how to support myself. Doctoring is what I know, and sometimes even love.

When Your Doctor Is a Jerk

Doctors fall prey to the same human failings and foibles that all of us struggle with, which means that some of us inevitably act like jerks. Whether from toilet training that went horribly awry at the age of two, or from being bullied at school, we doctors can have some personality issues. As a patient, you will occasionally encounter one who is seriously messed up.

How do you handle a jerky doctor? Well, if you need an unusual surgery and he or she is the best in the world for your particular condition, then I advise you to grin and bear it until your problem is handled. Otherwise, vote with your feet. And if you work with or for the aforementioned jerky doctor, you have a big decision to make.

Secret Doctor Fantasies

- The Nobel Committee arrives and presents us with the Nobel Prize in Medicine in the middle of a busy and stressful office day "just because."
- Diagnosing a rare disease that we've only read about in med school and no other doctor even considered.
- Being told "Doctor, you saved my life!" multiple times a day.

- Having our entire staff break out into applause when we walk into the office (this is a longer shot than winning the Nobel Prize).
- Not having any paperwork to do or labs to check for one full day.

What Makes Doctors Smile

- A child drawing us a picture, even when it's an utterly unrecognizable blob. "This is you!" they exclaim proudly, and we wonder if it's really been that long since we went to the gym.
- A grateful kiss on the cheek from an elderly woman who reminds us of our own grandmother.
- Someone losing weight, quitting smoking, or becoming cancer free.
- Going home to our families while it's still light outside.
- Having the feeling, however fleeting, that what we do makes a difference.

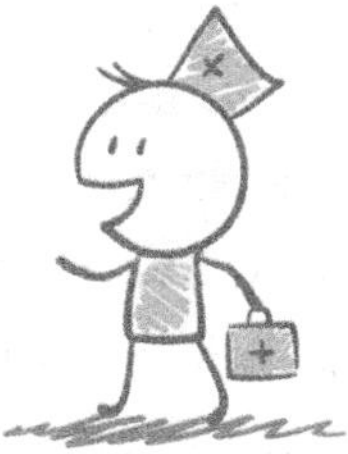

CHAPTER 11
SURVIVING YOUR INSURANCE COMPANY

THIS CHAPTER IS DESIGNED to help you see health insurance in a logical, sane way without resorting to potentially illegal activities involving a ninja suit and the cover of darkness.

It is vital that you understand what health insurance companies are for. Health insurance companies exist for two reasons:

1. To make money
2. See #1

In reality, that's why *every* for-profit business exists. A business that additionally helps its customers and employees enrich and improve their lives is a stellar one. That kind of business is a win-win situation. Every business should strive to achieve this.

But there's a big problem. The "product" that insurance companies sell is health, and even, arguably, life. These companies bridge the gap between patients and potentially lifesaving treatments, between people and quality of life. Unlike providing consumers a choice between, say, loaves of bread ("wheat, rye, white, sourdough, with or without raisins"), they offer a grisly selection ("would you like to live reasonably well for the two or three more years, or suffer a horribly disfiguring and/or painful demise in the next six weeks?"). Honestly, is health really *optional?*

Health insurance companies feel that in order to *make* money, they should *spend* as little of their money as possible. They try to accomplish this by enrolling healthy people in their plans, making them pay a bunch of money out of their own pockets up front, and encouraging them to stay healthy. This is a great system for the companies. Unfortunately it's not great for you, especially when you:

1. Are sick
2. Get sick

That's when the real "fun" begins.

Health care legislation is currently in force to help, but its long-term future is uncertain. No matter what permanently emerges as law, you can expect that health insurance companies will find creative ways of saving themselves money. They'll make their modest plans more expensive, or they'll offer limited benefits, or they'll seek to expand their markets to other countries that are less regulated, like the tobacco companies have already done. They might do all of these things and then some.

With more health care costs being shunted to consumers, the role of insurance is rapidly changing. No longer can you count on it to cover all of your medical expenses. Now its only real purpose is to keep you from being completely wiped off the map financially. I met one uninsured man who was previously healthy but had to have emergency surgery. The bill for his inpatient hospital stay was $111,000. That alone would be enough to make me physically ill; how about you?

Shopping for Health Insurance

I use the term *shopping* reluctantly, as most of us prefer to shop for things we enjoy, things we anticipate will bring us pleasure. Shopping for health insurance is like planning your funeral. Can you afford mostly catastrophic coverage (think of being mummified in bandages with your leg slung up in the air), or a regular HMO plan? Do you want an all-metal casket, or will a plain pine box do? It's just not pleasant.

As a physician, I thought I'd have no problems picking my own policy. I understand words like *deductibles* and *PPO.* I understand how HMOs work. But it turned out to be exactly like the time I ignorantly volunteered to watch a group of a dozen two-year-olds during a church function. Solo. All alone. "No sweat," I singsonged. "I know how kids work—I know exactly what to do!" I envisioned having a Wonderfully Fun Storytime, with their tiny faces in Rapt Attention, followed by an Idyllic Group Nap.

Hardly.

Someone fed those kids sugar cookies and Kool-Aid right before I got there—they were totally hyped up and ready for action (do you remember the movie *Mad Max?* If not, think of cage fighting). Over the next three hours, it was all I could do to keep them from killing each other. "Put the matches down, Jacob!" "No, no, Suzy—Becky's leg doesn't go in the toilet!" One sincere mother, on dropping her child off early that evening, told me to ensure that Little Johnny used the bathroom every hour or he would have an accident. "No sweat," I chimed. All I can say in retrospect is "Sorry, Johnny."

Back to insurance.

When I left government service, I had to buy my own health insurance. I was confident that a healthy nonsmoking person could get a fair rate. I envisioned years of reasonable premium payments, a doable deductible, and running blissfully in slow motion through The Golden Fields of Healthiness.

Hardly.

When I got my premium statement, it was twice as much as the online quote. It had exceeded my monthly car payment in size and was approaching the mortgage payment stratosphere. After an appropriate period of freaking out, I called the insurance company. They dryly assured me that I had selected the wrong plan "for my needs." I've since learned from that experience, and I submit for your consideration some important steps in selecting the right insurance plan:

STEP 1. Acquire the appropriate mindset.

Have you ever taken your car in for a simple oil change and known the standard "you should replace your air filter" sales pitch was coming? It's so very predictable. "Three . . . two . . . one" goes your mental countdown, and out comes the technician with this downcast, worried look, shaking his head, gently cradling your supposedly spent and useless filter close to his bosom like a wounded thing. You expect that. Or how about when you take your car in for repair? You go in expecting that you're going to pay a ton of money and quite possibly get ripped off.

I highly suggest that you view your dealings with health insurance companies the same way. Insurers like collecting premiums and dislike claims. They do not exist for your benefit—keep your expectations low. That way you won't waste time being incredulous over their heartlessness and can instead turn your precious energy into positive action.

STEP 2. Decide how healthy you are right now.

If you already know you're in poor health, skip the rest of these steps and just fork over your life savings, in cash, to the insurer of your choice—one that has a cool name might work well. If they balk at accepting a suitcase full of cash, offer to throw in boxes of chocolate and free back rubs for the underwriting staff. Hey, whatever works.

If you're reasonably healthy, you have a few more decisions to make.

STEP 3. Take a wild stab and guess how badly your health might deteriorate.

How much of your life savings can you gamble every year? $10,000? $5000? $3500? This is your deductible. With each passing year come more aches and pains, more suspicious moles on your skin, and more episodes of waking up not knowing where you are. Are you willing to allow these nuisances to slide by, knowing that you have to pay the majority of the bill yourself for each and every doctor's visit? "Not a problem," you say. "I'll just creep about very gingerly and avoid dangerous undertakings, like leaving the house." You obviously need a low deductible if you're broke. The only problem with this plan is that your monthly premiums will be much, much higher. And face it, you have to eat. Or do you? Skinny people get better insurance rates.

STEP 4. Decide if you need teeth, and/or the ability to see.

After you select the main body of your insurance plan, you will be asked if you'd like to fork over even more money for "add-ons," typically dental and vision coverage. It's very empowering to decide whether you prefer the basic dental plan, which helps you keep some of your teeth, or the enhanced plan, which gives you a 20 percent discount for keeping the rest. Ditto for your vision coverage. You're in the driver's seat, my friend. Unless you can't see to drive.

STEP 5. Decide if you want to become a hermit on a deserted island and not ever have to worry about health insurance again. Sharks yes, insurance no.

The Uninsured

There's a not-so-old urban legend about an uninsured man in Florida who urgently needed heart bypass surgery. Reportedly he committed a robbery so he could go to jail and be eligible for care. Obviously, I don't advocate crime as a way to get help. But so many people in our country are so very desperate. The inherent gross disparities of access to health care can no longer be ignored.

Case in point: Let's say I see a patient with weight loss and abdominal pain. She has excellent insurance, so I send her for a CT scan. The very next patient I see after her has the *exact* same symptoms, but she's uninsured. She needs the same CT scan, but simply cannot afford to pay thousands of dollars for it. A much-cheaper X-ray won't show me the organs I need to see.

Now what? Why doesn't she have the same access? Is she (gasp) not as important or worthy as the patient before her? Did the self-pay patient spend her time in high school goofing off and sleeping in detention, while the insured patient got straight A's? Ah—here's a good one: Is the self-pay patient a lazy, unproductive leech, and the insured patient an industrious, self-sufficient patriot?

These stereotypes are lies we've been subtly and consistently fed. The overwhelming majority of uninsured folks are extremely hardworking men and women. Some work two (or more) jobs to make ends meet. Some are self-employed business owners, logging crushing hours in their business every week. Health care and health insurance are just too expensive. Consequently, medical apartheid is alive and well in this country.

America is on the brink of a health care meltdown, and we're only beginning to ask questions as a nation that we should have asked long ago.

Is health care a right or a privilege? How much should tests cost? How much should doctors earn, and how should they be compensated? Do we really even need doctors anyway? Should people with bad habits like smoking and drinking receive any help? If so, how much? And so on.

Patients constantly ask me my opinions on the ongoing health care quandary. I tend to be dismissive, because a fifteen-minute office visit isn't even enough time for me to take care of their medical problems, let alone risk a lengthy rant. No one has any idea what will ultimately emerge as our "new" health care system. What I do know is that our current one is prohibitively expensive and fundamentally inequitable.

When You Don't Have Health Insurance

The Affordable Care Act (ACA) has helped insure many millions of uninsured and underinsured Americans. I've personally witnessed many patients who had been postponing much-needed treatment and surgery finally be able to access care and live healthier lives. There are many others, however, who still cannot afford the health care plans offered, and live in states where there are no subsidies to assist them. So they continue to go without.

Lawmakers are threatening to kill the ACA, yet have not provided alternative solutions to our chronic and worsening health care crisis. If this indeed does occur, what options do uninsured patients have?

Other sources of coverage, such as COBRA, Medicaid, and the Veterans' Administration, are available if you meet their eligibility requirements. Otherwise, community health centers (CHCs) can be a great source of less expensive medical care.

CHCs are real medical offices that are independent from county health departments; they are not "free clinics." These doctor's offices receive grants to provide primary care services in medically underserved communities, where the density of doctors is lower. Their fees are income-based and substantially lower than those of private practices. They may also have relationships with labs and hospitals for reduced rates on laboratory tests and radiology studies.

To pay back my medical school education, I traveled the country as a commissioned officer in the Public Health Service, providing medical care at various CHCs. Because I was a federal asset, the sites received an additional physician but didn't have to pay for one. The CHC doctors on staff at each site were consistently excellent and deeply committed to their patients. The clinical acumen my colleagues demonstrated was, without a doubt, comparable to physicians in private practice.

If you don't have insurance, CHCs are excellent options. They can be found online under "community health centers" in your particular geographic area. Good luck!

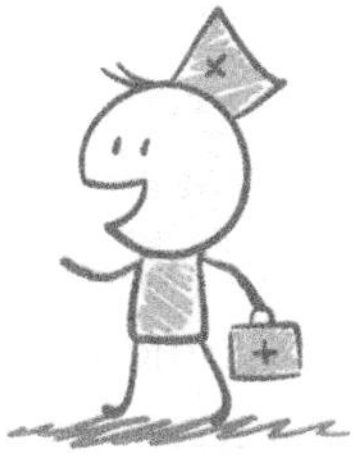

CHAPTER 12

MERCENARY MEDICINE

I got the bill for my surgery. Now I know what those doctors were wearing masks for.

—James H. Boren

Mercenary: adj. primarily concerned with money or other reward. Grasping, greedy, acquisitive, covetous, predatory. (Oxford Desk Dictionary, 2001)

When you go to the doctor's office, you fully expect to be the center of attention. It's *your* time, right? But these days the doctor may barely touch you, and you're whisked out before you've had the chance to tell her half of your issues. If you somehow manage to blurt out a few concerns, you may get a seemingly snotty reply that she can only handle one thing per office visit. Please don't take this personally. Most likely, your doctor is enmeshed in a system beyond her control. Or she's just mean. In that case, you might want to find a new doctor.

I once had a physical exam by a doctor who was billed as the head of his department. I try hard not to reveal that I'm a physician whenever I go for medical care, as I want to see how the doctors treat their patients under normal conditions. Several times I've had to blow my cover because things weren't going well, if you know what I mean. But I told this particular doctor that I was a colleague at the outset in order to save him time—he was quite busy that day.

This man proceeded to fill out my physical paperwork—get this—without even touching me. He didn't even lift his little pinky finger in my direction. There was no stethoscope taken out, no thoughtful examination of any kind. I even shared with him that I had a heart murmur, and apparently that failed to stir him to action except to continue to scribble in silence. I left the visit in awe. I wondered if I should report him for "medical nonchalance." This is not as bad as malpractice, but it might be on the same continuum.

This experience confirmed what many of my own patients had been trying to tell me for years. And I had never, ever believed them. They would share that their previous doctors had not examined them at all, or had only examined them in a cursory manner. This behavior is not right, and we cannot excuse shoddy medicine. But like I said before, we docs have issues. So the next time you're treated shabbily, try to be more understanding of the deep things that drive your doctor's strange behavior—and then find someone more well-adjusted to see.

So what is your doctor's problem anyway? In the grand old tradition of blame shifting, it's not (all) your doctor's fault, really! It's the lack of time. The same crunch of time experienced by the American worker has seeped into the medical profession. Did you know that many office-based physicians are under daily patient quotas? They are contracted to see a certain number of patients a day, are often rewarded for seeing more, and are sometimes penalized for seeing less. What this means is that your doctor typically has anywhere between five (if he is triple-booked) and fifteen minutes to hear your concerns, examine you, diagnose your problem, and come up with a reasonable, non-life-threatening treatment plan.

It's easy to see that not much serious disease can be stamped out in that miniscule amount of time. To the dismay of one of my previous clinical directors, it took me at least two of those precious minutes to say hello and engage in the normal pleasantries of human conversation. After an extremely enlightening conversation with my boss, in which we discussed the various benefits of me continuing to be employed, my new time-saving techniques were in full swing. For example, look at the difference between these two doctor visits:

Old Way of Seeing Patients

Barely Employed Doctor (smiling cheerfully): "Good morning, Mrs. Williams! How are you today? It's nice to see you—how is your husband Earl doing? Why don't you come up here on the exam table so I can examine you . . . take your time. Is that knee of yours giving you any problems lately? No? Then tell me about those blackouts and chest pain and bloody stools you told the nurse you were having." (Thirty minutes later . . .) "I'll see you in two weeks to go over your test results and to see how you're doing on the new medication. Give my best to Earl!"

New Way of Seeing Patients

Grouchy but Employed Doctor: "Okay, lady—get on the table, and make it snappy. Now look here—I'm only gonna deal with one thing. Pick whichever one is worse, I don't care." (One minute later . . .) "Take this pill. Now stop yer whinin' and get out!"

The latter scenario seems extreme, but at its core is a grim reality. How can patients comfortably relay their most intimate concerns and feelings when we physicians are slaves to the clock? How can physicians possibly be empathetic and good listeners when we're primarily focused on how far behind we are and how quickly we can exit the exam room? How can our current way of seeing patients *possibly* work?

Time management gurus give us docs tips on how to behave as if we're giving patients more time than we really have. We're told, for instance, that touching our patients gives them the perception that their visit was about four minutes longer than it actually was. So whenever your doctor touches you gently and empathetically on the shoulder, it might be a subtle clue that your visit is over! Just kidding. Take your touches wherever you can get them; they're therapeutic. But realize that your doctor may experience supervisory static and administrative consequences for not being brief with you.

Lest we should give an unbalanced picture, the time crunch also exists on the patient side of the equation. Over the last few years, I've seen more and more patients in a crazy rush to get out of the office. In our fast-paced, technology-driven culture, people simply want to get pills and get out. Some folks even schedule important, time-sensitive engagements (client meetings, transcontinental flights, weddings, etc.) immediately after their doctor's appointments, which inevitably run long (surprise!) because we find a medical problem in them or the patient ahead of them that requires attention. Also, a good 70 percent of my daily appointments are interrupted by patients' cell phones going off, particularly in the middle of Pap smears and prostate exams. If the doctor is rushing and the patient is rushing, how can that possibly be productive?

The Future of Medicine

When I share with my doctor friends where I believe the practice of medicine is heading, they find my musings unnecessarily alarmist and amusingly fanciful. I comfort myself with the knowledge that since the dawn of time, people who have advanced new ideas have been laughed at and dismissed as kooks. At first. Here's how I, the resident kook, believe the future will materialize.

Doctors Will Disappear

The natural world is ruled by money. As it goes, changes follow. Advanced practitioners, also known as physician assistants (PAs), nurse practitioners (NPs), midlevel practitioners, or physician extenders, are less costly to train and hire than physicians. Having these medical professionals on staff also allows patients greater access to care, and patients find their experiences with advanced practitioners effective and fulfilling. The scattered primary care physicians who remain in the next ten to fifteen years will likely be supervising office staffs of advanced practitioners, until advanced practitioners become licensed to practice independently nationwide.

Advanced practitioners are performing notably not only in primary care, but in the medical specialties as well. They serve with distinction in ICUs, operating rooms, and cardiac labs all over the country. Specialist physicians will be around a bit longer than their primary care colleagues, but likely they will also be sublimated over time. Medical school enrollment will contract with shrinking physician demand, while NP and PA schools will be bursting at the seams. Program mergers will be the rule. The medical school programs that survive will largely exist to train subspecialists and researchers.

I'm not bitter—this is simply the way business flows. This transition will probably take about fifteen to twenty-five years to complete. The primary care physicians who are currently in practice will be just fine unless they have to relocate and find a new job, particularly in an urban area. But those earnest young people who are considering becoming medical doctors now had better have a plan. When they're job hunting and find that most offices are seeking advanced practitioners, they should have another skill on the side, like plumbing, just in case.

However, this whole discussion will largely be moot, because:

Most Medical Professionals Will Be Replaced by Computers

Billions of people depend on computers every day. Computers cook our food, drive our cars, wake us up, inform us, and help us exchange ideas with the world. There's no escaping the onslaught of technology upon the human body. Our cell phones will soon measure and modulate our moods and decide which calls we should take or ignore. Computers are even amplifying our brainwaves to move objects in space. So is it so hard to imagine that computers will provide our medical care? They don't take vacations or demand benefits, they're much less prone to error, and they don't need sleep. Okay, sometimes they do get a little cranky and crash, but unlike humans, they can usually be repaired without comparable bother or expense.

Remember the handheld TriCorder device in the classic *Star Trek* television series? Dr. McCoy just scanned people and diagnosed what was wrong. In a similar vein, I want you to imagine a booth. Let's call it the HealthPro 3000, and let's say you have a cold. You walk inside the booth, sit down, close the door, and get comfy. You insert your insurance card and any required cash (of course) and then click off your symptoms on the computer screen with a light pen. Next, the machine takes digital pictures of your face and throat, and you insert a flexible fiber-optic tube with disposable tips in your ear to check for ear infection. This could also be used to tickle your throat for a strep test. If you have a rash, another device with a disposable cover could be rolled over the rash.

The computer displays a printable diagnosis and patient care instructions, then electronically forwards any needed prescriptions to your local pharmacy (or dispenses simple drugs itself) and bills your insurance company. If anyone develops one of these machines after reading this book, I fully expect a 5 percent cut. Thank you.

"Oh, great," moan the pharmacists. "The machine would even take *our* jobs." Sure. Especially when everything in life is distilled down to the almighty dollar. A computer doctor might be less helpful for Pap smears and rectal exams (yikes!), but those more invasive procedures could still be performed by humans. My point is that *fewer* humans will be required.

Does this shock you? It shouldn't.

"But Dr. Woodhouse," you protest, "what about the sacred relationship between the doctor and patient?" Well, thanks for asking, but it's slowly dawning on me that most folks with non-life-threatening medical issues really don't *want* an intimate relationship with their physician. What they want is a quick and accurate diagnosis, rapid and safe treatment, and rapid recovery. Patients with more serious conditions like cancer require that personal touch and ongoing follow-up, so the few remaining specialists will take care of those folks.

However, as the human-computer interface deepens and broadens, the need for mental health professionals will also increase. Psychiatrists, psychologists, priests, ministers, counselors, masseuses and others will flourish as people become more connected to the digital world and more disconnected from themselves and from God. But at least some health care professionals will have a job.

"I'll never give up my primary care doctor!" you say. Well, when all your insurance company will pay for is a trip twice a year to the HealthPro 3000, we'll see. You might even like the machine better! At least when it recommends you stop smoking or lose weight, it won't have a superior, condescending attitude unless it's programmed that way.

See? That wasn't so fantastically paranoid as you thought, right? Bottom line for both patients and health care professionals: The future is coming. Be prepared.

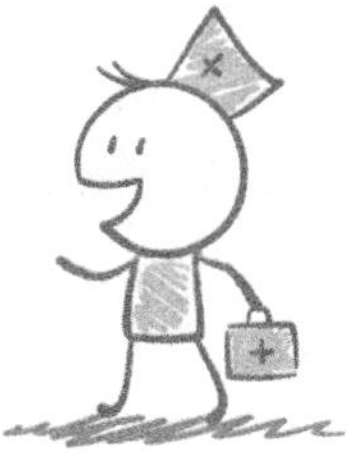

epilogue

FINAL ADVICE FOR A GREAT LIFE

I have told you these things, so that in Me you may have perfect peace and confidence. In the world you have tribulation and trials and distress and frustration; but be of good cheer [take courage; be confident, certain, undaunted]! For I have overcome the world. [I have deprived it of power to harm you and have conquered it for you.]

—John 16:33, Amplified Version

ALL THROUGHOUT THIS BOOK, I've shared my opinion on a whole bunch of stuff, and this chapter is no exception. I challenge you to read the whole of it even though you may be of another faith, or have no faith, or have given up on faith years ago. Your life could be at the precipice of total transformation if you do. The words quoted above were spoken by Jesus to each and every human being, and I invite you to consider what these words could mean to you.

Why Your Spirit Matters and Why Doctors Should Care

Human beings are composed of spirit and soul (mind, will, and emotions) housed in a body. Our spirits represent our most fundamental essence, and they deeply affect our souls, how we think and feel. It's logical that problems on the inside can manifest as symptoms on the outside. So when a doctor ignores a patient's spirit as if it didn't exist, she may unwittingly truncate the healing process.

Insomnia, anxiety, depression, and constant pain and illness despite normal results on thorough serial evaluations: All are potential examples of medical problems which may stem from underlying "soul holes." Soul holes can arise from wounds inflicted by others or come from deep unmet needs or emptiness. This is critical for physicians to recognize, because pitching pills into soul holes may provide limited treatment of symptoms, but it will not provide any lasting cure. Once the pills run out, the symptoms reoccur.

After years of practice, I've found that no pill, no diet, no supplement, no fitness regimen, no seminar, and no amount of positive thinking can decidedly and with finality cure patients of soul holes. Lasting cures can only occur at the spiritual level. Otherwise, patients are never completely free. They resign themselves to an impotent captivity, claiming, "This is just the way I am." Not so. You were not meant to live in bondage.

Soul holes exist in everyone, manifesting themselves in different ways and in varying degrees. No one can function with holes on the inside, so people attempt to fill them themselves. And many resort to sinister, self-destructive means to do so.

MY STORY

I was born the only child of a military family. We moved around a lot. But my parents lovingly provided a safe haven for me within the bosom of our little family. Sheltered, introverted, and bookish, I focused contentedly on my schoolwork and geeky after-school activities like Yearbook and French Club. I even lettered in varsity badminton! I had few friends, and I didn't date. But I didn't care. I was an excellent student. Life was safe and full and good. And God? I had a vague notion that there was a God somewhere up there, but that was about it.

Life acutely worsened when I left home for college. Bereft of my sheltered family life, I was exposed to a new, dark world. And although I successfully fled from drugs, alcohol, and blatant debauchery, I was totally unprepared for the daily, bitter assaults to my self-esteem. I was surrounded by other really smart kids. Many were from wealthy families and were much more worldly and better traveled than I. What made me different? What made me special? Was I pretty? Was I interesting? Would anyone want me? Why would they? Who was I? *I had no idea.* I was dazed and confused and desperately lonely. I longed for emotional security and acceptance but was instead riddled through and through with gaping, yawning soul holes of insecurity and inadequacy.

Predictably, I was an easy meal for the first predator who crossed my path. He threw me a meager shred of attention, and in my deranged condition, I clung feverishly to him. From college through medical school, I allowed this man to verbally abuse and disrespect me—all so that I could feel wanted! But fake love is destructive. My soul holes widened and deepened with each passing year.

Over the next four years of residency, other so-called boy "friends" arrived. They were battling with their own soul holes, manifested in alcohol dependence and pornography addiction. And they were losing their battles. The longer I stayed in relationship with these men, the more spiritually ruined and emotionally impaired I became. I was lonelier than ever before. However, as a resident, I was simply too busy for a breakdown. I ignored my gaping soul holes. I buried my pain deeply in my work. I told myself I had more important things to attend to, such as completing my residency and not killing anyone in the process.

I graduated residency and got a job in a new state. Although I was well prepared for doctoring, I was ill prepared for a contented life. I was earning good money, but an unshakable emptiness dogged me. Insecurity, self-doubt, guilt, and shame riddled my daily thoughts. My life lacked true love, power, and purpose. I felt like I was dying inside. And I was. That's when I did something radical.

Who Needs God, Anyway?

There are many things in life I'm not sure about. I'm not sure if I will ever get over my love affair with food or how many more years I can squeeze out of my furnace. But I am absolutely, 100 percent certain that you experiencing your very best life ever is completely dependent on one thing.

And that one thing is God.

Wait—not THAT God—not the one with the flyswatter and lightning bolts just ready to smite you whenever you mess up. And definitely not the old doddering one who sits idly by while evil runs rampant, throwing his hands up in feeble resignation.

No, your best life involves the all-powerful, all-knowing, and very present God of everything, who is good, perfect, just, wise, and more beautiful, if we had eyes to see Him, than we could ever imagine. He made you, knows all about you, and loves you unconditionally. He really, truly wants to be your heavenly Father, your Dad.

Wait—not THAT dad—not the one who rejected, abandoned, or abused you growing up. Not the one who was physically at home but emotionally unavailable. God is the kind, merciful, encouraging, strong dad you've always wanted. If you had a fine human father, God wants to be even better to you, and even closer to you, than that.

You might ask, "If God is so good, has unlimited power, and wants to love on me, why has He allowed such hurt and pain in my life and other people's lives? Why hasn't He intervened?" That is the eternal question, isn't it? The answer is that He *is* intervening—He's always intervening; but in ways we cannot see. Evil is in the world. Through our fallen nature, humans hurt and harm one another. Sickness and death are part of our reality. The fact that our lives are broken is not God's fault. But know this: He will certainly judge evil and restore all things to their original, perfect state. And typically, His intervening has less to do with reversing your negative circumstances than it does with getting you smack-dab face-to-face with Him.

The most critical problem is this: We're all separated from God relationally because we've all ignored or flat-out rejected the very notion of God and His authority over everything. We've tried to go our own way and often suffered greatly for it. Left to our own devices, we're powerless to be anything but devil bait.

Why Jesus Is Absolutely Critical

None of us is perfect. But God is. Totally. So on our own, we can't even dream of getting close to Him—our imperfections and failures keep getting in the way. But Jesus ingeniously provided a way for us and God to be completely reconciled. Jesus was born a human baby, but with God's DNA—that's why a virgin birth was necessary. He grew up and lived a perfect life as a real man here on earth so He could both identify with our human plight and represent us before God. Then He took the full punishment that is legally due as a result of our thumbing our noses at godly ways to think and act. That punishment, frankly, is death, both an eternal physical and spiritual separation from God.

Crucified on the cross, Jesus took all of our messes physically upon Himself in order that we might possess His righteousness in a free and clear exchange. For many agonizing hours He became a thief, a liar, a murderer, a child molester, an adulterer, an alcoholic, an addict, a wife beater, a prostitute, a thug, a white-collar criminal, and every other broken form of human you can imagine. *All* of humankind's possible sins were represented in Him. "But I'm none of those awful things," you might say. Sure, but have you ever told a little lie? Have you ever said an unkind thing or even had an unkind or impure thought? Every single one of us has. None of us can claim absolute moral perfection. But Jesus could.

If we choose to accept what Jesus did for us on our behalf, we can freely run back into God's arms because our sins are totally erased. And Jesus not only removed all our sin, but also all the guilt, all the shame, and all the condemnation that came with it. We can now have a clean slate before God, without fear or dread of punishment. We're free to be our real selves before Him. He's free to reveal to us who He really is and not who we've imagined Him to be. That's it. It's not complicated. We can never, ever earn God's approval by trying to be good or do enough good deeds! On our own, every single one of us will always fall short somewhere. Jesus's sacrifice is a totally free gift. All we have to do is accept it.

But Jesus did not simply die as a human martyr. As God's divine Son, Jesus had the power to not stay dead. He had the power to resurrect Himself and stay alive for the rest of eternity. In the same way, He has the power to make humans who believe in Him alive eternally. As strange as it may sound, there's life beyond the one you're living right now. Your body will age, get old and wrinkled, and die. But that's not the end of you. Heaven is real, perfect, and gorgeous, and is lovingly prepared for those who have a real relationship with God. And hell? This is not a fire-and-brimstone book, and fear is never a good basis for any love relationship—I don't believe in scaring people into considering Jesus. But hell is real nonetheless, and it is a very bad place. Why live in hell on earth, then die and go there unnecessarily, just because we never got on the same page with God?

The Radical Thing I Did

In the midst of my descent into emotional hell, I looked up and found myself surrounded. My resident buddies and even my hairdresser were all Christians. On Sundays they'd attempt to drag me to church. I felt incredibly inconvenienced and bored by the whole idea. In my opinion, Christians were mindless drones who had no free will and who didn't have a lick of fun. I sporadically complied just to get them off my back.

I wish I could say that I went to church and "got saved." I did not. Instead I got bombarded with fake religiosity that left me persistently unhelped. I learned church lingo, got spit on by frenzied preachers, and even started tithing to try to get on God's good side. I had no inkling of who God really was, or of who I was, and I continued to spiral downward.

So what did I do when I finally realized I was a complete and total wreck and needed help? I picked up my barely used Bible and blew the dust off. Somehow it opened to the book of John, and I began reading.

It was *wonderful*. I felt as if light were shining out from the pages onto my face! I'll never forget that moment. I had reached the critical point of desperate hunger where I could hear God. I read about Jesus' life, what a real life lived in fellowship with God looked like, a life where there was no room for fear. I read about the intense, unconditional love that God had for me through Jesus' sacrifice. Even after totally blowing it, even when I had made a complete mess of things, God *still* loved me enough to give me the way back "home."

I was floored. Even at almost thirty years old, my life could be rebooted! I was important to the One who really mattered—important enough to die for. And there was nothing I could do to deserve His love. The supreme God of the universe was lovingly reaching out to me, talking to me, even when I didn't deserve anything at all from Him.

Why? Because a long time ago Jesus decided to love me by standing in the gap between me and God, despite all of my warts and messes and issues. And I decided to accept His gift.

On that day I became a real Christian—despite myself—and I have never been the same. Jesus took up permanent residence in my heart, and promised to never vacate the premises. My soul holes are definitely getting filled. I still have challenges and bad days; being a Christian doesn't exempt me from making mistakes, feverishly grasping at old ways of coping, or having problems. But with Jesus, I have all the supernatural help and hope I could ever ask for—and then some. Even my challenges have been tailor-made to accomplish God's grand and good purposes for me.

There's an extraordinary, life-changing little book entitled "He and I" by Gabrielle Bossis, a 20th-century mystic who recorded the intimate conversations Jesus had with her towards the end of her life. In the journal, Jesus Himself speaks about the awesome new relationship every single one of us can have with Him:

"In Me you can find everything: all the love you need to help you. So don't be afraid of making use of the One who loves you so. Don't you come

to Me with more confidence than to any friend on earth? Aren't you at home in My heart? It should be that way too, since for each soul I am the unique, the incomparable One."

—April 20, 1941

"I am the One who makes whole. So give Me your wretchedness. Show it to Me with your two hands like a beggar. I said to the apostles, 'It is I, don't be afraid.' Such gentle, loving words! And I say them over again to you."

—June 19, 1941

"At-onement, do you understand what this means? This is life, all of it. Nothing else counts. Offer yourself unceasingly to our oneness, and My action will be even greater. Even if this were your only way of praying, your life would show no ordinary mark but one that is altogether supernatural and precious in the Fathers' sight."

—April 16, 1942

Given all these fantastic things, I just can't lose. How's that for the best life ever?

WHAT ABOUT YOU?

When you make the quality decision to accept Jesus, God gives you a new identity, which actually ends up being the full expression of who He created you to be in the first place. You will still be "you," but brand-new!

When you accept Jesus for real, you are saying to Him, "You can take over. I'm done trying to manage everything. I give You full rein to do what You think is best for me. And I will do what You desire that I do, no matter what." No small task. But God will help you to both *want* to submit to His lordship and to get it done. The rewards will be phenomenal, both on earth during your lifetime and in heaven for all time. You and those God placed around you will never be the same. Your life will change drastically for the better, either suddenly or over time—God knows—as you make the most important decision of your entire life. Will you reject Jesus as made-up, illogical nonsense, or will you consider and accept Him?

All you have to do is believe in Jesus, who God sent to rescue you from you. Believing simply means trusting Him, listening to Him, and doing what He says to do (which always turns out to be your best plan anyway). That's it. Jesus makes it pretty easy for you to have a brand-new life firmly rooted and grounded in Him. You never have to be afraid, because He is in control. Even if the world whispers otherwise in your ear, you matter greatly because God made you specially, personally. He wants you here on earth right now; He wants you to receive His love and give Him love back. It only takes a real yes from you. That's what it took for me—a *real* yes.

Saying Yes

When you say yes to God, He will graciously give you a meaningful life, filled with power to accomplish the purpose for which He made you. You won't have to strive anymore to make your life count, because He will lead you step-by-step into the fullness of your real life, the one He's always intended you to have. He will give you a joyful life, filled with a growing love for Him and for your fellow man. And He will give you a pure life, filled with new, divine power to say no to unhealthy ways of thinking and living. He'll change your heart, your mind, your desires, and your eternal destiny forever. Are you willing?

If you're willing, tell Him so. If you mean it, God will hear you—no doubt. He'll make the miracle happen: the exchange of your old messed-up life for your new life in Jesus. If you let Jesus lead, He will take you places you could never get to alone.

Lord Jesus, come into my heart.

I confess that I don't have all the answers. I've missed it, I've blown it, and I need Your help. You're the only One who has the power to make my life right.

I turn away from my sin—all my mistakes and failings—and I turn to You.

I believe You are the Son of God and that You died to take away my sin. You rose from the dead and are alive in me right now, listening to me.

I don't understand all this right now, but I believe that You will make Yourself known to me as I reach out to You.

I release control of my life and hand it over to You. You know best how to handle it anyway and will give me the real life I was meant to live. Please fill me with Your Spirit so that I can hear Your voice.

Thank You, Lord Jesus, for being Lord of my life. Amen.

If you said that prayer, *congratulations!* The Bible says all the angels in heaven are throwing a huge party over you right now because you have now been adopted into God's family. You may not *feel* that you are different, and your desires may not change instantly. But if you truly meant what you just said, an eternal transaction has surely been made that can *never* be broken.

What Do You Do Now?

First, get a study Bible written in modern English. That way you won't be needlessly stumbling over "thees" and "thous." *The Life Application Study Bible* in the New Living Translation (NLT) was my first Bible. *The Message* and the Contemporary English Version (CEV) Bibles are also easy reads. The Bible is God's love letter to you. You might want to start in the book of John as I did, because there you can really see God's love for you in action. Read a little bit every day. Get to know Jesus, the One who traded His life for yours. What was He like? How did He handle the hard places in His own life?

Make it a priority to spend quality time alone with Him every day. After all, how can we know someone intimately if we don't spend any time with them? Talk to Jesus about anything and everything that's going on with you throughout the day, thank Him for all that He does for you and gives you, and tell Him how awesome He is. This is called prayer. Your prayers never have to be fancy or sound like somebody else's prayers. Keep it simple. Jesus knows all, sees all, and even knows what you're going to pray before you open your mouth. His help desk is open 24/7 for life technical assistance, including guidance, comfort, requests, and thanksgiving!

Next, be sure to be quiet and *listen*. Wait to hear His voice, which is often very quiet. Then do what He says to do without delay, doubt, or fear. The more consistently you do this, the more intimate the two of you will become.

Don't walk alone. Find a friendly church that believes in Jesus' divinity, teaches the Bible, and encourages you to read it for yourself. Going to church does not make you right with God. That's all Jesus. Going to church does not substitute for spending time alone with Jesus and reading His instructions. But it *should* help you get to know God better, practice loving and serving others, and celebrate the reality of God with other believers. Surround yourself with Christian mentors and friends who will challenge you to grow.

Lastly, keep your mind focused on your earthly and eternal futures, which are good and full of hope.

Below are some Scriptures about your new identity in Christ. It's a powerful new identity—that's why they call this the "Good News"!

So now there is no condemnation for those who belong to Christ Jesus. And because you belong to Him, the power of the life-giving Spirit has freed you from the power of sin that leads to death. (Romans 8:1–2, NLT)

Anyone who belongs to Christ is a new person. The past is forgotten, and everything is new. (2 Corinthians 5:17, CEV)

You have accepted Christ Jesus as your Lord. Now keep on following Him. Plant your roots in Christ and let Him be the foundation for your life. Be strong in your faith, just as you were taught. And be grateful. Don't let anyone fool you by using senseless arguments. These arguments may sound wise, but they are only human teachings. They come from the powers of this world and not from Christ. God lives fully in Christ. And you are fully grown because you belong to Christ, who is over every power and authority. (Colossians 2:6–10, CEV)

And, as Jesus said in "He and I":

"And I'll bless you, because you will at last have responded to My call...the call of the One who

stood at the door listening to the life stirring in the house, and wondered whether it would welcome Him or not. For if He stands outside waiting, it is because He knows that He may be driven away. Sometimes they don't even want Him to wait. They say, 'Never will You come under my roof.' As though He were an evil-doer, He who died for love of them…But when they say, 'Come in, and stay with us,' then this poor, lonely One knows the joy He describes as 'His delight to be with the children of men.'"

—Sept. 21, 1940

Please contact Poema if you'd like to share your decision with us. Let us celebrate with you!

Peace to you,
Catherine Woodhouse
Poema Enterprises, Inc.
Email: info@laughableadvice.com

Made in the USA
Monee, IL
04 November 2026

67387018R00115